Routledge Revivals

Language Assessment for Remediation

Published in 1981, this book describes and critically examines the standardised tests and modes of assessment available and most commonly used by speech therapists, psychologists and educationalists.

Tests and other assessment procedures are discussed and therapeutic strategies suggested. Thus, psycholinguistic approaches such as ITPA, the Reynell Developmental Language Scales and the Aston Index; linguistic techniques such as LARSP and phonological assessments are described, and adult disorders as well as childhood problems, are reviewed. There is also a brief consideration of the problem of assessing the language of those not speaking English as a first language.

The book serves as a core text for student speech therapists and also as a reference for those practicing or researching in speech therapy, special education and linguistic pathology.

Language Assessment for Remediation

David J. Müller, Siân M. Munro and Christopher Code

Routledge
Taylor & Francis Group
ROUTLEDGE REVIVALS

First published in 1981
by Croom Helm Ltd

This edition first published in 2018 by Routledge
2 Park Square, Milton Park, Abingdon, Oxon OX14 4RN
605 Third Avenue, New York, NY 10017

Routledge is an imprint of the Taylor & Francis Group, an informa business

Publisher's Note
The publisher has gone to great lengths to ensure the quality of this reprint but points out that some imperfections in the original copies may be apparent.

Disclaimer
The publisher has made every effort to trace copyright holders and welcomes correspondence from those they have been unable to contact.

A Library of Congress record exists under LCCN: 81166236

ISBN 13: 978-0-8153-7963-8 (hbk)
ISBN 13: 978-1-351-21530-5 (ebk)

Language Assessment for Remediation

David J. Müller, Siân M. Munro and Christopher Code

CROOM HELM LONDON

Croom Helm Ltd, 2-10 St John's Road, London SW11

British Library Cataloguing in Publication Data

Müller, David J.
Language assessment for remediation.
1. Handicapped children – Language – Testing
I. Title II. Munro, Siân M.
III. Code, Christopher
401'.9

ISBN 0-7099-1706-6
ISBN 0-7099-1707-4 pbk

CONTENTS

PREFACE

Overall, this is meant to be a practical book. Consequently, we have directed it at individuals who have a professional interest and who are taking, or intend to take, responsibility for implementing language remediation. It is aimed at practitioners and in particular speech therapists, but is likely to be of relevance to teachers as well as educational and clinical psychologists. The book has been written with students of these professions in mind and can be described as an introduction to the field.

Assessment we feel is far too often discussed in isolation from remediation, whereas to us they are intricately linked. Bearing this in mind, the main aim of writing the book was to review a variety of procedures available to assess language and to examine their usefulness in guiding remediation. In preparing the book we have had to select from a vast number of specific procedures which are currently available, but in doing so we have tried to represent the range of different approaches.

In discussing remediation we have deliberately refrained from being prescriptive and instead have reviewed the variety of techniques relevant to the assessment procedure under discussion. We hope that this approach will help readers make up their own minds and by following up the suggested references and sources enable them to select the techniques most appropriate to their own requirements.

It may be that in this book we have posed more questions than we have provided answers. This might not be a bad thing, if we have also been able to show that assessment alone is not the answer to any question concerning the remediation of language.

1 LANGUAGE, INTELLIGENCE AND REMEDIATION

Chapter Outline

The role of language in intellectual functioning is discussed. It is argued that in order to remediate deficient intellectual performance, special emphasis needs to be given to language and this naturally involves the accurate assessment of linguistic behaviour. Three standardised intelligence tests are evaluated in the light of their success in diagnosing language deficiencies. The suggestion is put forward that although of value in identifying potential language difficulties, these tests are of limited use in making diagnoses and in suggesting remediation. It is concluded that intelligence tests need supplementing with other measures specifically designed to identify and remediate deficient language performance.

Introduction

It is almost impossible to discuss intellectual behaviour without referring in some way, either explicitly or implicitly, to the role of language. Yet, there has been little agreement concerning the exact nature of intelligence and Pyle (1979) begins an excellent text by noting that even after years of investigation and debate, there is still no consensus on what intelligence actually is. This has led to considerable uncertainty concerning the best way in which to assess intellectual activities in order to implement remediation.

Despite this uncertainty, it is beyond dispute that children and adults engage in activities which are termed intellectual, and that in doing so they use language a great deal of the time. In fact Viaud (1960) has argued that from an evolutionary perspective language has acted as the dividing line between specifically human ways of thought as compared to those ways which are common to man and animals.

Consequently, where it is intended to remediate intellectual behaviour, it is almost impossible to do so without recourse to language. At the simplest level, therapists are almost certain to work through the verbal medium, and it is likely that the treatment itself will be directed at various forms of linguistic activities and involve quite complex procedures. This means that in order to plan and implement effective remediation, careful consideration must be given initially to the role of language in intellectual behaviour.

Language and Intelligence

Discussion of the relationship between language and intellectual development, has often centred around the debate of whether language precedes and hence is causal in the development of thinking, or if it is simply a means of representing what is already known. The former view owes a great deal to the seminal Soviet work of Vygotsky (1934) which was not translated into English until 1962. This is in contrast to the Genevan school led and dominated by Piaget and his co-workers (see for example Piaget, 1968; Sinclair-de-Zwart, 1969). The practical value of this debate is unclear, but an extremely lucid review of the theoretical viewpoints and related research has been undertaken by Cromer (1974).

However, Bruner (1975) has put forward a solution to this problem which seems to have the greatest therapeutic potential. He has suggested that at times language is causal and 'moulds' an individual's thinking and that at other times language acts as a 'cloak' encompassing and representing what has already been learned. Implicit in this argument is the view that the relationship between language and thought is determined situationally. Developmentally, it appears reasonable to assume that as children mature they learn to utilise language in ways which are most appropriate to their intellectual activities.

Consequently, the debate concerning whether language precedes thought or thought precedes language, is of limited value to those with an interest in remediation. It is clear that language interacts with and influences intellectual behaviour in two main ways. First, language is more often than not the medium through which an individual's ideas or thoughts are made public and hence serves an important representative function. Secondly, in a variety of situations, language initiates and refines the thinking process and enables new ways of perceiving the world to emerge. In serving both these functions, language is without doubt a major influence in intellectual behaviour, and it is almost impossible and of little therapeutic value to conceive of language without thought or thought without language.

This suggests that in order to remediate intellectual functioning, it is important to consider these particular functions of language. In particular, careful attention must be paid to assessing language in order to diagnose the problem and hence plan remediation. A starting point is to examine how successfully standardised tests of intelligence measure language and to see whether they provide sufficient information to suggest reasons for any deficiencies.

The Stanford-Binet Intelligence Scale (1960)

The Stanford-Binet has undergone a number of revisions since its inception by Binet at the turn of this century. The version currently in use is the 1960 revision (Terman and Merrill) which is suitable for children aged from 2 to 14 years. There are also four adult scales. In the age range 2-5 years, children gain one month towards their mental ages for each subtest correctly completed, whereas from the age of 5 years they gain two months. Hence six subtests represent each half year in the first part of the Scale and a year in the second part.

This procedure of gaining credits in the form of months results in intelligence being stated in terms of a mental age. Hence, a child of 6 years who is able to complete as many subtests as might be expected of a 7 year old, would have a mental age of 7. This meant that in designing the Scale, the subtests had to be arranged in order of difficulty rather than by content and had to reflect what children might be expected to do at given chronological ages. Therefore, the mental age score reflects overall intellectual functioning rather than specific abilities and the IQ (Intelligence Quotient) score which can be attained from the mental age score is related to general performance.

In order to give an indication of the range of abilities assessed by the Scales, Sattler (1974) has classified the subtests according to their content. He has suggested that seven areas are assessed as follows: language; memory; conceptual thinking; reasoning (verbal and non-verbal); numerical reasoning; visual motor skills; and social intelligence. Furthermore, factor analysing the subtests suggests that there is a heavy loading on verbal production and verbal reasoning. This is supported by an analysis of the number of subtests reflecting verbal skills. Approximately one third of the subtests can be classified as assessing language ability or verbal reasoning in some way.

From a therapeutic perspective, the assessment provided by the Stanford-Binet tends to be more descriptive than diagnostic. Many of the subtests involving language, assess knowledge of vocabulary including identifying parts of the body, recognising pictures and defining the meaning of words. Other subtests assess verbal abilities such as eliciting opposites or explaining differences between various items. There is little emphasis given to an objective assessment of verbal production and more stress is placed on the skills of comprehension.

In conclusion, although the Stanford-Binet enables language performance to be described in such a way that general problems can be noted, it has limited therapeutic implications. From the subtests alone, it is difficult to explain why children may be having difficulties and hence the Scales are of limited diagnostic value. But perhaps the greatest difficulty in using the Stanford-Binet to assess language is that the subtests are arbitrarily distributed. Whereas at the age of 2½ years at least four subtests assess language, at the age of 4½ years it can be argued that there is only one subtest relating to language. This makes it almost impossible to assess fully language at all the age ranges. These two factors make it difficult to use the Stanford-Binet as a guide for remediating deficient language performance.

The Wechsler Scales

David Wechsler has been responsible for producing a series of tests designed to assess intelligence. There are three tests readily available; the Wechsler Pre-school and Primary Scale of Intelligence (WPPSI) published in 1967 for use with children aged 4 to 6½ years, the Wechsler Intelligence Scale for Children (WISC) revised in 1974 (WISC-R) and for use with children aged 6 to 16 years 11 months, and the Wechsler Adult Intelligence Scale (WAIS) published in 1955.

All three tests have a similar format, being divided into a verbal scale and a performance scale. Each scale has up to six subtests. This format makes it possible to calculate separate verbal and performance IQs as well as providing an overall measure of intelligence. The concept of mental age used in the Stanford-Binet has been replaced by the use of a deviation intelligence quotient. This is obtained by comparing each subject's test performance with the scores earned by others in their own age group, rather than with the complete age range for which the test is designed. Wechsler (1974) has argued that this approach produces more meaningful results.

The verbal scale is designed to measure those abilities which are based on previously learned verbal material and are to a large extent dependent upon experience. It consists of the following subtests: information (general knowledge); comprehension; arithmetic; similarities; vocabulary; and short term memory of digits. The performance scale is intended to measure immediate problem solving ability and relies less on the recall of past experience and more on practical expertise in novel situations. It consists of the following subtests: picture completion; picture arrangement; block design; object assembly; and coding or mazes. Most of these are timed and bonus marks awarded for quick performance.

At a therapeutic level it would appear that the Wechsler Scales are particularly useful in identifying specific language deficiencies. Using the scales it is possible to compare any individual's verbal score with their performance score and their overall general intelligence. Furthermore, discrete subtest scores can be compared and profiles of their overall abilities built up. In the case of dyslexic children for example, it has been shown by Thomson and Grant (1979) that they score lower than controls on Information, Digit Span, Arithmetic and Coding, but higher on Object Assembly and Picture Completion.

However, the diagnostic value of the Wechsler Scales is not as clearly evident as might be expected. The main difficulty in using them to assess language, is that it is questionable whether the subtests of the verbal scale are comprehensive. Most of them appear to measure only receptive language skills without testing for any understanding of grammatical forms. A second and related problem is the question of whether or not all the verbal subtests actually tap language ability. It is questionable whether remembering a list of digits or doing mental arithmetic are really tests of verbal ability. Similarly, testing for general knowledge is not really assessing language ability.

Therefore, although the Wechsler Scales measure verbal and performance abilities separately it can be argued that the subtests used to assess verbal ability are of little diagnostic value. There are similarities with the Stanford-Binet in that, although both include assessments of language ability, neither are sufficiently comprehensive or specific to give a clear indication of the therapeutic procedures which can be adopted.

The British Ability Scales

Elliott, Murray and Pearson (1978) designed the British Ability Scales to assess a wide range of capabilities for the age range 2½ to 17 years. The Scales are unique in that they have been standardised on a British sample using criterion referencing which allows each individual's performance to be assessed in relationship to a particular ability, rather than with a sample of the population. This approach is based on a statistical procedure called Rasch scaling.

There are twenty-four separate subtests or scales altogether, including some which assess traditional school-based abilities. It is possible to calculate IQ scores by administering only four of these scales, separate combinations having been specified for three broad age ranges. The scales are grouped according to the underlying processes being assessed as follows: visual-motor speed; reasoning; spatial imagery; perceptual matching; short-term memory; and retrieval to facilitate the application of knowledge.

A number of these processes are considered to have a verbal component of varying degrees. Three out of four of the scales assessing reasoning rely on language: those of formal operational thinking and social reasoning are presented verbally, and the scale assessing knowledge of similarities is based on verbal items. Two of the scales assessing perceptual matching include copying or matching letter-like designs and the third involves finding objects after receiving verbal descriptions. For over half of the scales assessing short term memory the mode of response is verbal.

However, the most detailed assessments of language ability are grouped under the process of retrieving and applying knowledge, where five out of seven scales have an obvious verbal component. A test of naming vocabulary designed for children aged 2½ to 8 years assesses the ability to name objects presented pictorially. There is a scale to test verbal comprehension for the same age range which involves carrying out various actions in response to verbal commands. There is a test of verbal fluency designed for children aged 4 to 17 years to assess the creative use of language. Finally, there are two tests of reading and defining words, for children aged 5 to 14 and 5 to 17 years respectively.

This wide range of scales measuring language is far more comprehensive than the assessments included in either the Stanford-Binet or Wechsler scales. Using the British Ability Scales it is possible to assess knowledge of vocabulary, comprehension skills, production skills (creative and non-creative), reading levels and the ability to reason verbally. Furthermore, it is possible to select scales which measure specific language abilities as required.

However, it can be seen that like the tests previously mentioned, the British Ability Scales are only indicative of a problem and are not really diagnostic in the sense of highlighting specific disabilities and suggesting therapy. They appear to describe quite accurately what children are capable of, given certain tasks, but they do not fully explain the reasons behind any individual child's performance. Knowing that a child has a limited vocabulary or has difficulties in reading does not in any way guide the therapist towards possible therapeutic techniques, despite being able to identify the problem. In conclusion, it does not seem that the British Ability Scales are of any more practical value in guiding remediation that either the Stanford-Binet or Wechsler scales, although such a conclusion may be rather premature at this stage and should consequently be viewed with caution.

Conclusion

Although definitions of intelligence rarely include specific reference to language it is implicit in most viewpoints that language plays a major role in intellectual behaviour. This is reflected in the range of abilities assessed in traditional intelligence tests, all of which include items specifically designed to assess language. Thus by using intelligence tests it is possible to get a clear indication of how well an individual is able to perform on tasks requiring the use of language. In this sense they can be viewed as *screening tests* which enable attention to be focused on individuals identified as having distinct language problems.

However, rather than simply describing and identifying a problem it is of value in guiding remediation to employ a diagnostic approach towards assessment. There are at least three stages in this process. First, the problem must be identified and it has to be shown that it can be attributed to the relationship between language and intellectual performance. This can be seen as the *screening* stage where an attempt is made to identify individuals at risk. Intelligence tests are able to fulfil this function with a considerable degree of reliability.

The second stage is to attempt to *describe* any deficient language performance as accurately as possible in order that the specific problem can be identified. Intelligence tests meet with varying degrees of success at this stage. The most comprehensive test discussed in this chapter is the British Ability Scales, from which specific subtests can be selected as required. However, there are considerable limitations in the descriptive capacity of the British Ability Scales. By themselves the Scales do not really provide sufficiently precise descriptions of the language behaviour under investigation nor is it possible to generalise from them to include areas not specifically tested. It may simply be, for example, that an individual's poor performance on comprehension is purely test specific and may not be repeated on a different test. Taking the second stage overall, it can be concluded that although intelligence tests meet with some success in providing descriptions of the behaviour in question, considerable limitations are more evident.

The third stage is to try and make a *diagnosis* which in turn suggests either one or more *therapeutic strategies* which might be implemented and evaluated. In other words the tests used need to generate possible reasons for poor performance. Circular arguments such as the notion that a child has poor language ability because of low intelligence, give no indication of possible approaches towards remediation. It is at this stage that intelligence tests are of less value. Even the British Ability Scales give very little information to assist the therapist in implementing treatment. Furthermore, intelligence tests are of even less value at this stage for use with adults suffering from acquired language disorders, due to the difficulty of estimating intelligence prior to the onset of their problem.

This distinction between description and diagnosis will become an important theme in this book. Remediation depends not only on recognising and describing the problem, but more importantly on being able to make a prognosis and providing some indication of the therapeutic strategies which can be implemented and evaluated. The following chapters will examine this in more detail, concentrating on those approaches to assessing language which have more direct implications for therapy than would be gained from using intelligence tests.

2 EVALUATION OF PHONOLOGICAL AND GRAMMATICAL ABILITIES IN CHILDREN

Chapter Outline

Six of the most frequently encountered tests and techniques for assessing phonological and grammatical development are discussed. The review of the technique relating to phonological processes highlights the work of one American and one British author. Of the remainder, the EAT and LARSP are British tests, and the Goldman-Fristoe Test of Articulation, the Developmental Sentence Analysis and the Carrow Test for Comprehension of Language are American. The above are evaluated with particular reference to their effectiveness as bases for the planning of remediation.

Introduction

As we have seen, the previous chapter has endeavoured to describe the relationship between language and cognition. Claims for such a relationship have led to a situation where tests measuring aspects of cognitive development are frequently administered to children with language disorders. This is particularly the case where the language problems are thought to result from general difficulties with representational behaviour. Even in these cases there is a need to look also at the actual structures uttered by the child. This need for a linguistic approach becomes increasingly apparent when dealing with specifically linguistic disorders.

In both cases, linguistics can provide not only a convenient method of description but also 'a principled procedure' (Crystal, Fletcher and Garman, 1976, p. 109). Such a procedure entails the organisation of language data according to specified criteria (such as levels of complexity) which in turn imposes structure on a remedial programme. The developmental characteristics of tests such as those described below are an attempt to provide this structured framework.

The Edinburgh Articulation Test (EAT)

Theoretical Background

This test, published in 1971, is intended to give a picture of the developing phonology of young children, at least with respect to consonants, the articulations of which are felt to provide a reliable indication of overall speech mastery. Attention is not given to vowels as they are established in speech at a very early age. Anthony, Bogle, Ingram and McIsaac (1971) claim that the EAT presents a 'balanced and comprehensive picture of consonants and consonantal clusters occurring in English at various positions in the word structure in monosyllabic, disyllabic and a few polysyllabic words' (see page 3 of Test Manual for details of positions included).

The EAT has been standardised on a sample of 510 children from varying social backgrounds. Three years is the lower age limit as the attention of children below this age is considered unreliable. The upper age limit is established at 6 years because it is at this point that articulation reaches a near approximation to that of adult speech.

In order to obtain numerical data plus detailed information about the child's phonology, the EAT is presented in two sections.

(a) *Quantitative Analysis*. To provide a compact test, a few members of a phonological group are selected to represent the whole. For example, only certain representatives of the 'plosive + r' group (/br/) are included as it was established that all members of this group followed the same developmental trend. Owing to the limited attention of many pre-school children, elicitation of utterances takes the form of a naming game, the resulting single words purported to fulfil the following criteria: that they
   (i) are familiar to the children;
   (ii) give maximum phonological information, e.g. 'garage' provides details of word-initial /g/, word-medial /r/ and word-final /dʒ/;
   (iii) discriminate, in terms of difficulty, between normal and speech retarded children.

(b) *Qualitative Analysis*. Here, the items of the Quantitative Section are regrouped according to phonological similarity 'so that groups of sounds requiring remedial treatment may be more readily identified' (Anthony and McIsaac, 1970, p. 154). For instance, the first four words 'milk, chimney, spoon, tent' include nasals. Furthermore, the Qualitative Section is assembled under six headings (see 'Description').

This enables the child's responses to be located along a continuum so that results can be examined for patterns of development. The authors argue that young children's articulations rarely fall into neat right/wrong categories, as there are dialectal and developmental factors to be considered.

Description and Administration

The Quantitative Assessment Sheet (see Figure 2.1) provides a space alongside each word for the phonetic realisation of the child's response and another in which to place a mark denoting in/correctness of each response.

Correct items are totalled to give a raw score which, by means of a conversion table, yields a standard score. The suggested 'danger level' is a standard score of 85 or less, pointing to a need for more detailed investigation of the errors. The table can also provide an 'articulation age', the 'danger level' being an articulation age one year behind a child's chronological age. A set of coloured pictures is provided, with one illustration per word. Repeated 'answer-words' and guessed responses are considered to be as valid as spontaneous responses.

The phonetic realisations are then transferred to the Qualitative Sheet, each realisation being assigned to one of these six columns: Adult form (extreme left) – Minor Variations – Almost Mature – Immature – Very Immature – Atypical (extreme right), thereby giving a visual lay-out of the child's articulatory achievement. Examples of the errors typical of each column are given on the sheet and are grouped vertically within each column to denote equal status in maturation. For example, under 'Almost Mature' substitutions for word-initial /sp/ are grouped thus – [s̪p] [s̡p] [s̢p]. The criteria adopted for this grouping are frequency of occurrence and phonetic similarity. These are important for they may be used when locating on the sheet any realisations not already exemplified.

Therapeutic Implications

The Quantitative Section of the EAT, described by Anthony *et al.* (1971) (p. 34) as 'a rather basic numerical assessment' offers only limited information on which remediation can be planned. The phonetic representations of the child's productions are more useful than mere scores, but as the authors include in the test only certain members of each sound group this information is somewhat restricted.

While it is true that the Qualitative Section gives additional perspective it nevertheless relies on the phonetic data gathered from the

Figure 2.1: Edinburgh Articulation Test/Quantitative Assessment Sheet

Name ______________________ Sex ______ Test given by ______________________

Address ______________________ Place of Test ______________________

Date of Birth ______________________ Date of Test ______________________

monkey	ŋk	sleeping	sl	finger	f
tent	t		p		ŋg
	nt	wings	ŋz	thumb	θ
fish	ʃ	garage	g	watch	w
train	tr		r		tʃ
umbrella	m		dʒ	string	str
	b	aeroplane	pl		ŋ
	r	spoon	sp	three	θr
	l		n	teeth	θ
milk	m	toothbrush	θbr	pencil	p
	lk		ʃ		ns
stamps	st	red	r		l
	mps		d	yellow	j
queen	kw	bottle	tl		l
clouds	kl	birthday	rθd	sugar	ʃ
	dz	horse(ie)	h		g
Christmas	kr	feather	ð	Indian	n
	sm	elephant	l		d
	s		f		j
bridge	br		n		n
	dʒ		t	matches	tʃ
flower	fl	soldier	s		z
chimney	tʃ		ldʒ	scissors	z
	mn		r	desk	d
smoke	sm	glove	gl		sk
	k		v		

Source: Reproduced by special permission from *Edinburgh Articulation Test* by A. Anthony, D. Bogle, T.T.S. Ingram and M.W. McIsaac.

Quantitative Sheet and is therefore also limited to a small number of types per token. It is difficult and unwise to attempt a treatment plan to include, for example, fricative phonemes, when one only has information about one word-initial [f], one word-final [s] and so forth.

However, there are facets of the Qualitative Analysis which have more positive implications for remediation. First, it is designed to distinguish between two types of problematic speech development, delayed and atypical, each of which is related to a group of specific principles and techniques. For instance, the structuring of remediation programmes for children with delayed phonological development tends to be based on what we know of the developmental progression in normal phonology. Secondly, the Qualitative Analysis can be used to identify speech patterns which are associated with different areas of pathology, such as high frequency hearing loss. Once again, the identification of a type of problem implies a particular approach or approaches to remediation.

Related Research

Using the EAT, Johnson and Somers (1978) investigated the question of spontaneous versus imitated responses in articulation testing. Having studied the behaviour of 64 normal 4 and 5 year old boys and girls, they concluded that there *was* a significant difference between the two modes of test presentation. Others (e.g. Siegel, Winitz and Conkey, 1963; Paynter and Bumpas, 1977) investigating normal and speech defective children, found no significant difference, a fact which has resulted, in some cases, in the adoption of imitative ability as the only mode of appraising a child's phonological development. This procedure has serious drawbacks for there are certainly clinical cases which demonstrate differences on imitated as opposed to spontaneous utterances. Thus, in omitting one of these modes of testing one is restricting an area of possible diagnostic and therapeutic significance. For instance, the techniques for working with a child who can imitate sounds will differ in some respects from those needed for the child who cannot imitate and requires help on articulatory placement and multi-sensory feedback.

An interesting paper by Somers (1979) described the design of a computer package for analysing data from articulation tests, the EAT being used as the data base. The output was in seven sections which included an item by item comparison of test and target data, statistical feature analysis, phonological processes, a table of realisation of target phonemes, and matrices of phoneme contrasts. This detailed type of information is potentially useful for the planning of remediation for it rapidly provides several types of analysis from a single set of data. This enables the clinician to pinpoint quickly the specific areas of weakness in the child's phonology and plan remediation accordingly.

However, Somers did point out the drawbacks of using a reduced data base such as the EAT. For example, he felt that the table of realisation of target phonemes would be much more meaningful and useful were it not for the large number of gaps resulting from the use of the EAT.

Appraisal

Anthony *et al.* (1971) describe their test as one of phonological maturation, but as a phonological approach which will 'bring out the pattern-forming capabilities of the elements of utterance' (Abercrombie, 1967, p. 71) the EAT is open to criticism. Hence, Grunwell (1975, p. 33) claims that it provides no direct information about 'the phonological contrasts operating in the child's language by comparison with the adult system'. This means that apart from the fact that the limited number of items restricts the phonetic information available, the EAT also provides little direct information on the child's ability to use sounds to signal differences in meaning.

Although the classifications of the Qualitative Analysis are useful as discussed earlier the criteria which determine these classes are not always clear. This is particularly so where the atypical substitutions are defined as being of two types, one of which is labelled 'childish (possibly purely very immature) substitutions'. Furthermore, as the authors' findings have been based on data collected from a normal sample of children, the realisations of the clinical population tend to be missing from the columns of the Qualitative Section. The EAT's structure is said to be open-ended so that phonetically similar realisations may be fitted into the basic structure, but it can be difficult to decide on the correct column location of some children's forms.

The emergency level derived from the Standard Score of the Quantitative Analysis has its uses, but such a score offers no guidance as to therapeutic strategies. Nor does the Qualitative Section provide clear principles upon which remediation methods can be selected and constructed. It does, however, provide a model of normal articulatory maturation which is helpful in continuous assessment.

Goldman-Fristoe Test of Articulation (GFTA)

Theoretical Background

Like the EAT, this (American) test aims to provide a systematic means of assessing an individual's articulation of consonants and consonant clusters. Most of the single consonants of English are tested, those omitted being of infrequent occurrence in the language. Although not designed to study vowel production, all vowels and most diphthongs are present so that 'deviations' can be noted.

Another similarity with the EAT is the condensed type of articulation testing where the examiner has to listen for more than one sound per word. This method is based on the theory that the resulting reduction of stimulus words minimises the time taken to administer the test, and prevents the subject from losing interest, while maintaining a high level of information.

However, the GFTA is different from the EAT in that it samples both spontaneous and imitative production, and includes both single word and conversational speech production. The authors claim that this test thus has 'the diagnostic potential for comparing articulation at different levels of complexity . . . providing the examiner with a method of determining the locus of greatest difficulty and of judging the stability of articulation . . .' (Goldman and Fristoe, 1972, p. 7). In order to sample these levels, the GFTA is divided into three sections, the Sounds-in Words, Sounds-in Sentences and Stimulability Subtests. The rationale underlying the last two sections mentioned is of particular interest:

(a) *Sounds-in Sentences Subtest*. Previous methods for testing connected speech are not considered representative of the type of spontaneous (non-imitated) production occurring in everyday conversation. This subtest is therefore intended to elicit 'content – controlled, conversational-type speech' by means of story-repetitions (but is limited to those consonants most likely to be defective).

(b) *Stimulability Subtest*. The assessor requires information about the sounds most readily responsive to remediation, so this subtest is designed to test the subject's ability to produce a previously misarticulated phoneme when given maximum stimulation.

The GFTA tests phonemes in word-final, -initial and -medial positions. Although this classification has been criticised (see 'Appraisal'), the authors claim that since articulation defects vary with the positions of the phonemes, they should be assessed in these positions.

Description and Administration

(a) *Sounds-in-Words Subtest*. This is similar to the EAT in that each child is required to respond spontaneously to pictures at a one-word level. These responses, of which there are 44, provide information on sounds, whenever possible, in all word-positions. Whole words are not phonetically transcribed. The response matrix is set out so that phonemes used earlier in speech development appear at the top and later developing sounds below. Thus, stimulus words contain phonemes located at different points on the matrix, involving the assessor in much scanning in order to record responses where designated, e.g. 'house', /h/ is located on the fifth line of the matrix and /s/ on the twenty-fifth. Scanning is aided by utilisation of a number and colour coding system.

(b) *Sounds-in-Sentences Subtest*. Using sets of pictures as a guide, the child is required to recount two stories read aloud by the assessor. The stories are printed on the Score Sheet so that the child's realisation of each assessed phoneme can be quickly and easily recorded at the relevant points in the text. The realisation can be transferred to the response matrix later, aided by the coding system. Again, transcriptions do not involve the total word structure.

(c) *Stimulability Subtest*. Those phonemes mispronounced in (a) are assessed here, at syllable, word and sentence levels, in that order. Each misarticulated phoneme is presented to the child for imitation and a note made of his response. If the phoneme remains incorrect, multiple stimulation is given. The child again imitates and the response chart is marked accordingly (see p. 14 of manual) before proceeding to the next level.

Percentile rank norms for (a) and (c) are provided for errors by age from 6 to 16+ years of age, although the illustrations and words, on the whole, are suitable for younger children. These norms were obtained from the errors produced by children on the GFTA during a National Speech and Hearing Survey on a stratified sample of 38,884 children.

Therapeutic Implications

The Sounds-in-Words and Sounds-in-Sentences matrices provide a picture of the word positions in which misarticulations most frequently occur, but these tend to lead to a type of remediation based on phoneme position, for example, correction of initial, final then medial

/s/. Such an approach obscures processes such as assimilation which may have caused the misarticulation.

An impression of the most frequent type of error (omission, substitution, distortion) can be gained from these matrices. Some of these errors will relate clearly to general strategies adopted by the child, for example, 'stopping' of /s/ to [t] or /m/ to [p]. Other errors will be due to processes not immediately apparent from the matrices, such as omission of sounds resulting from weak syllable deletion. Therefore, if the clinician wishes to relate therapy to the organisational principles of the child rather than correcting individual sounds, the Goldman-Fristoe is of variable assistance.

Of course, it must also be borne in mind that the inclusion of only one token per sound-in-position type gives a narrow view of the stability of the child's phonology. The child whose matrix errors are truly representative of a consistent, long-standing difficulty presents with different therapeutic needs as compared with the child whose misarticulations on the test belie the fact that the phoneme can be produced correctly. The latter inconsistencies may well point to a phonological patterning problem as opposed to one of mechanical sound production.

The Stimulability Subtest is important for planning remediation for it gives information on the child's ability to produce misarticulated sounds correctly with auditory and visual stimulation and at varying levels of complexity.

Related Research

Using the Sounds-in-Words and Sounds-in-Sentences Subtests of the GFTA, Johnson, Winney and Pederson (1980) compared the production of 35 articulation impaired children on picture elicited single word (SW)- and connected speech (CS)-sampling methods. Comparisons were made of the two testing conditions with respect to the number and type of errors on each.

The results revealed marked differences between the two sampling methods, which included a greater number of total errors on CS testing with defective phonemes not identified on the SW sample. Qualitative differences were also noted, such as CS yielding a greater number of omission- than substitution-errors but the reverse being the case for SW testing. Johnson *et al.* concluded that remediation planning should, therefore, be based on CS sampling and analysis.

The primary focus of Elbert and McReynolds' (1978) study was the role of context in promoting generalisation of correct speech sounds. Five children who substituted [θ] for [s] were trained to produce /s/

correctly in three syllables and the generalisation patterns were analysed. To qualify as a subject a child was required to produce errors on the phonemes /s/ and /r/ in three tests, one of which was the Goldman-Fristoe.

The authors found that variables other than context played an important role in the generalisation displayed by the child, one of these variables being stimulability (as assessed on the Goldman-Fristoe subtest). They felt that scores predicted correct production of /s/, which suggests that a critical factor in this area of remediation may be the development of the ability to imitate.

Appraisal

Some of the drawbacks of the Goldman-Fristoe Test have already been discussed in the section on therapeutic implications. Most of the criticisms result from the three-position format of this test which is essentially word oriented. Of course, it could be argued that words do not appear as separate entities but as a sequence of syllables. Thus McDonald (1964) suggests that an adequate articulation test should consider articulation as a series of overlapping movements, and does not feel the articulation of single words to be truly representative of a child's abilities. Admittedly, the Sounds-in-Sentences Subtest attempts to move into the realms of continuous speech but the usefulness of this approach is hampered by the adherence to phoneme-in-position analysis, the assessor being required to select out only *single* phoneme realisations for the matrix.

The search for possibly significant relationships between a particular phoneme and the others in its environment could be facilitated by the Goldman-Fristoe Sampling procedure which allows for the analysis of several phonemes per test word. However, this does not apply to every word included. Of the 47 target words on the Sounds-in-Words Subtest, 22 are intended to provide information on only one phoneme, for example,

pajamas – medial /dʒ/
or chicken – medial /k/

Furthermore, the search is rendered difficult and lengthy by the location of originally proximate phonemes on different parts of the matrix, for example the /b/ of 'rabbit' is on line 6 while the /r/ is on line 17.

Overall, this test could be said to provide phonetic information which, in itself is useful, but it is not able to provide a real insight into the phonological patterning of child speech.

The 'Phonological Processes' Approach

Theoretical Background

The field of study concerning the part played by 'processes' in phonological acquisition is both complex and controversial. As such, only introductory statements are possible within such a general chapter on assessment.

In the past, studies of normal phonological development tended to *describe* the child's output, but nowadays there is a concentration on determining the rules behind that output. Many of these more recent studies claim that, in attempting adult target words, children adopt organisational principles that govern the patterning of their speech. These are referred to as 'phonological processes' which are said to simplify the child's output, for example deletion of unstressed syllables:

Target: 'banana' [bəˈnaːnə]
Child's realisation: [ˈnaːnə]

The term 'organisational' suggests that the child plays an active role in phonological acquisition, but there are those who disagree, considering the role to be a passive one. For instance, Smith (1973) suggests that children merely 'filter' the adult words without imposing their *own* structure on them.

Despite such differences of opinion, research into normal speech development is largely committed to the search for this rule-based behaviour and forms a foundation for studies of phonological disability. For example, workers such as Ingram (1976) and Grunwell (1977) have adopted the processes approach in examining abnormal phonology, where general stages of acquisition provide some framework for assessment.

Ingram stresses the active involvement of the child in assimilation and accommodation of the phonological input (adult sound system), implying that the child has an independent 'system' which gradually approximates to the adult model. There have been several arguments for (see Ferguson, 1968) and against (Stampe, 1969) the existence of a child's own system, but these are too lengthy to be reviewed here. The relevance of 'system' to assessment will, however, be referred to in following sections.

Description and Administration

It is important that the assessor obtains a representative sample (see

Ingram, 1976, pp. 76-97 for details on methodology of data collection), of a child's phonology, but this can be a difficult, time-consuming task. One should, however, ensure that the phonetically transcribed sample contains both spontaneous and imitated utterances and several items per sound.

Subsequent analysis of the child's simplification processes can distinguish between delayed and deviant phonological development in a manner described by Ingram as follows:

(i) use of processes which are the same as younger, normal children, i.e. delay;
(ii) use of the same processes as the normal but not in the same way, i.e. deviance;
(iii) use of 'unique' processes (usually in combination with some normal processes), i.e. deviance.

Table 2.1: Examples of Some of the Normal Processes Referred to in (i) and (ii) Above

Processes*	Examples	
Assimilation	'Dog'	[gɔg]
Cluster Reduction	'Spade'	[peɪ]
Weak Syllable Deletion	'Giraffe'	[ra:f]
Stopping	'This'	[dɪt]

*These and other normal processes cited by Ingram and Grunwell are essentially the same though classified somewhat differently.

Table 2.2: Examples of Some Unique Processes Referred to in (iii) Above

Processes	Examples
Lateralisation	'Sing' [lɪŋ]
Nasalisation	'Yes' [mɛ]
Initial Consonant Adjunction	'Empty' ['dɛpi]

In discussing the analysis of phonological processes, some consideration is due to the system resulting from the child's application of those processes. Delayed acquisition, for instance, implies a system similar to that of a normal (though younger) child, while the unusual use of common processes results in a deviant system. In Grunwell's (1977) investigation of 'phonological disability', following her description of processes appearing, the speech of each subject is analysed 'as an independent phonological system' (see 'Appraisal'). Grunwell (1980) gives a clear account of the processes effecting simplification of structure as opposed to those affecting the system.

Grunwell (1977) does not attempt to distinguish between different levels of processes (i.e. perception *v* production) as does Ingram. Also, she does not subscribe to the technical notational conventions utilised by Ingram and questions the degree of insight provided by such a sophisticated framework.

Therapeutic Implications

The implications discussed below are general and somewhat tentative. As pointed out in the previous section, phonological simplification processes have been observed in both delayed and deviant speech development, but it is not possible here to detail the specific needs of each. Rather it is intended to give a broad idea of the strategies available, leaving appropriate selection to the clinician.

While there are children with phonetic problems who would benefit from direct training of isolated sounds, we are more concerned here with those who can articulate most or all of the phonemes but are unable to pattern them within a linguistic framework. Analysis of the phonological processes used by this latter group indicates that they affect entire classes of sounds, implying that remediation should not be concerned with one phoneme at a time. Ingram (1976) advocates a focus on several sounds within a class because this has a wider effect than teaching an individual sound affected by several processes.

As the phonological simplification results in homonymy which reduces the contrasts in the child's system, the aim of remediation could be described as the elimination of homonyms leading to more effective use of contrasts and consequently increased intelligibility. Establishing which processes have the most detrimental effect on intelligibility provides a systematic method of deciding which processes to eliminate first.

If this is difficult there are alternatives. The occurrence of processes in normal speech development has implications for clinicians, for they can structure the remediation programme to begin with those processes most characteristic of young children. Alternatively, Ingram (1976) suggests that one first selects the optional processes which occur only occasionally as these should be the easiest to eliminate.

This emphasis, which is essentially on the *production* of phonology, does not imply that remediation should be based on repetitive sequences or increase of motor abilities. Since phonological production is thought to involve 'active organisational processes' (Leonard, Schwartz, Folger and Wilcox, 1978, p. 414) remediation work should be made meaningful for the child by illustrating continually how phonology operates within the total linguistic structure.

Related Research

Hodson (1978) investigated a model of phonological intervention for use with children whom she variously defined as having 'severe functional articulatory . . .' or 'phonological disorders'. She considered the one-phoneme-at-a-time approach to be inefficient for these children and described an alternative strategy already tried with 36 unintelligible children. This model involved suggestions for working in/directly on phonological processes as well as the development of areas such as word-final consonants and awareness of stridency.*

In the first of the three stages Hodson mentioned the development of back/front contrast as a means of dealing with the velar fronting process. However, in discussing regressive voicing assimilation (for example, 'card' > [ga̤:d]) she stated that voicing (and devoicing) was not a criterion for success at this stage of remediation.

Stage 2 included work on the awareness and production of stridency. Also, the simultaneous stimulation of the continuancy feature was possible since several sounds in this group of stridents were also continuants. The intention was 'to promote generalisation to other continuant phonemes, resulting in overall reduction of the stopping process' (p. 238).

Hodson concluded that this model allowed for the facilitation of phoneme production across processes (or features) which resulted in the children 'rehearsing' their newly learned productions before deciding on their final target.

Stoel-Gammon's (1980) paper presented a phonological analysis of four Down's Syndrome children aged between 3.10 and 6.3. This analysis included a description of their errors in terms of phonological processes. The author noted marked similarities in the use of processes between retarded and young normal children. Although this study did

* The feature (strident) is a property of sounds such as (s) which 'permit the airstream to pass through only a narrow opening in the centre of the vocal tract' (Sloat, Taylor and Hoard, 1978, p. 86).

not refer to remediation as such, its findings were relevant for they strengthened the feasibility of using the organisational strategies of normal phonological acquisition as a yardstick for designing programmes for the mentally retarded.

Appraisal

The comments made here are confined to the very basic concept of phonological processes, and there is no discussion of additional details and variations, such as Ingram's division of processes into optional and obligatory (see Cruttenden, 1977 and Dodd, 1978 for more detailed reviews).

One of the advantages of a processes approach to abnormal phonology is that it has the potential to explain what initially may appear to be random errors. Furthermore, processes reflect a set of systematic strategies, an awareness of which is far more useful as a basis for remediation than a purely phonetic description of the child's speech. While providing a more explicit picture of the simplifying characteristics in child phonology this approach avoids rigid formality.

It is an approach which enables the comparison of the child's realisations not only with the adult model but also with the realisations of other children. Nevertheless, Grunwell (1977) feels that it does not provide a total description of a child's patterns; she also advocates 'internal' analysis of the data as an independent phonological system.

This type of 'process' analysis has proven to be particularly useful in working with phonologically disordered children. These frequently display both delayed and deviant phonological patterns in the absence of intellectual, hearing or neurological impairment. However, the approach can also be applied to the assessment of children who *do* display such underlying problems of retardation, as discussed previously, and hearing loss (Oller, Jensen and Lafayette, 1978).

Language Assessment, Remediation and Screening Procedure (LARSP)

Theoretical Background

Crystal, Fletcher and Garman (1976) choose to concentrate on analysis at the grammatical level of language. While they refer to morphology in places, their main concern is with the other subfield of grammar, syntax, showing bias in the direction of production rather than comprehension. The 'centrality' of syntax to remediation appears to be one reason for its selection, another being ease of applicability, arising from the high degree of agreement existing between various syntactic studies.

The authors do not attempt to measure the lengths of sentences or utterances as they suggest that length is a value easily affected by too many variables. Furthermore, length reveals little of the complexity of an utterance. Also avoided is an 'all-or-none' scoring technique, which is seen as too inflexible and 'does not allow for the varying degrees of grammatical completeness' (p. 13). Nor is it the aim of the analysis to provide labels for linguistic disturbances. Such classifications are often vague and are considered, at the present stage of our knowledge of syntactic disorders, to be less useful than a comprehensive description of each individual's output. This need to be comprehensive is highlighted as one of the central goals of any work on remedial syntax, the other being the need for awareness of system. Comprehensive and systematic procedures, it is argued, are essential for objective, consistent analysis.

Comparisons with normal development are claimed to be inevitable when analysing a syntactic disorder. While the relevance of the normal sequence of development is arguable with regard to planning remediation of language disorders, it is felt that a linguistic profile is arbitrary unless related to the framework provided by developmental norms. An indication of the structures appropriate to various stages of development (see Chapter 3 of Crystal *et al.*, 1976) enables the assessor to pinpoint those structures the child has or has not acquired, both kinds being important in planning remediation.

The LARSP framework is based on the grammar described by Quirk, Greenbaum, Leech and Svartvik (1972) because it gives a comprehensive account of contemporary English. Also, its organisation into levels and the relationship between structural elements at certain of these levels (notably clause level) provides a 'direct and economical description of the data of syntactic disability' (Crystal *et al.*, 1976, p. 39).

There is a quantitative aspect to this description. All structures used by the child are counted so that an impression is gained of those structures used frequently and those rarely occurring. The purpose of these *raw* figures is to provide a ready indication of progress or regression.

Description and Administration

As seen in Figure 2.2 the Profile Chart is divided into two parts, the top quarter composed of Sections A, B and C, contains synchronic information, while the remainder is developmental.

Section A enables the assessor to eliminate problematic utterances thus ensuring the continuity and rapidity of the analysis. The large grid

Figure 2.2: Profile Chart

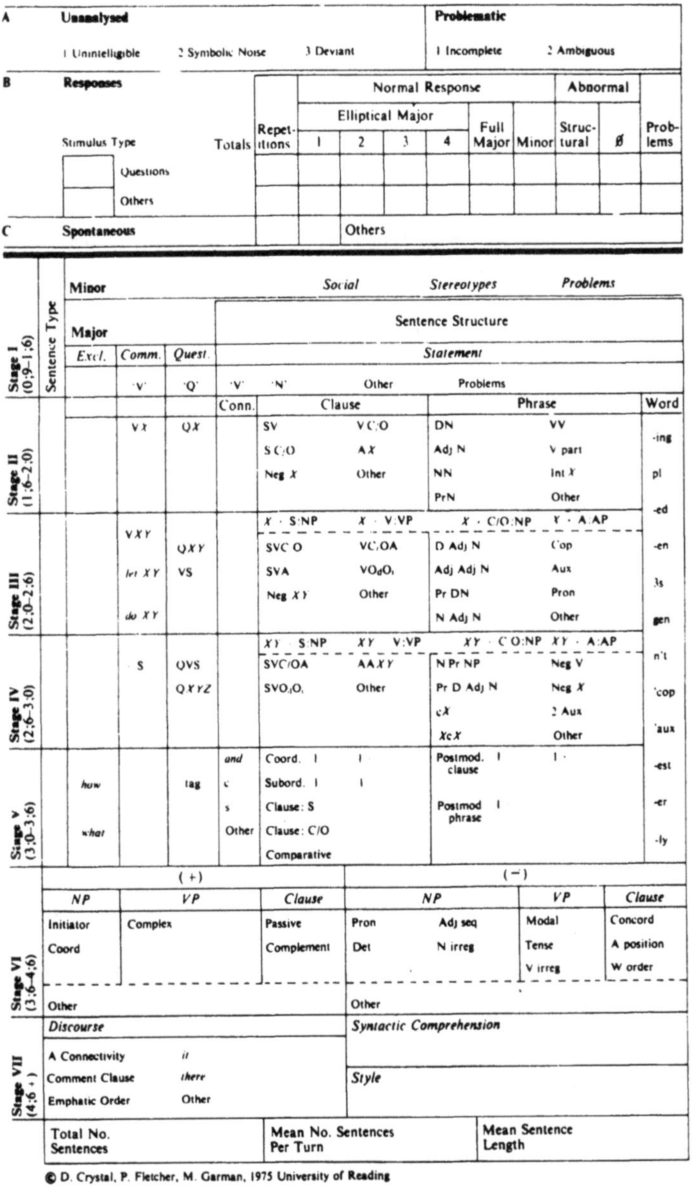

Source: Reproduced by special permission from *Language Assessment, Remediation, and Screening Procedure* by D. Crystal, P. Fletcher and M. Garman. Copyright 1976. Published by Edward Arnold.

to the right of Section B is self-explanatory, and the smaller grid on the left seeks to establish the proportion of spontaneous to response sentences. Section C presents a further breakdown of the numbers of spontaneous sentences, the main distinction being between self-repetitions and novel utterances.

The following points relate to those aspects of the Developmental Section which may not be immediately apparent:

(i) the Minor and Major sentence types of Stage I refer respectively to absence or presence of Subject-Predicate Structure;
(ii) the symbols appearing throughout this Developmental Section denote various grammatical elements, for example, Pr. D. Adj. N. > Preposition + Determiner + Adjective + Noun;
(iii) the stage of 'system completion' (VII) assesses the development of patterns ((+) features) never or partly utilised previously. It differs from previous stages because as the child, by now, is able to do a great deal that is syntactically correct, *errors* (or (-) features) are also analysed;
(iv) Stage VII includes analyses of syntactic comprehension and style, which do not contain examples of typical patterns as it is not yet possible to classify them in a precise manner.

Ideally, the data for this analysis should be obtained from a 30 minute sample of spontaneous speech, tape-recorded in two 15 minute parts, the topic of conversation in one part being the immediate environment, and in the other absent situations. It is possible, however, to curtail the sampling in order to lessen the time needed (see Crystal, 1979).

As soon as possible after recording, a transcription is made of the conversation, incorporating information on prosody, context and voice quality. Details of transcription conventions are available from both references given above.

The authors suggest that the data are then scanned several times, each scan having a particular aim:

Scan 1 determines the figures for Section A of the Chart (see previously);
Scan 2 relates to Section B;
In Scan 3, sentence connectivity is analysed;
In Scan 4, analysis of co-ordination, subordination,etc. takes place;
Scans 5, 6 and 7 are used for analysis of clause – phrase – and word structure patterns respectively;

In the 8th, the problem utterances resulting from Scan 1 are examined using knowledge (about the child's utterances) acquired from the other scans.

Therapeutic Implications

Language development is associated with maturation in spheres such as cognition and perception, which is why therapists have resorted to cognitive and perceptual training in order to remediate developmental language disorders (see Chapter 3). There are, however, children who have an 'independent' language problem who do not seem to benefit from such training. Crystal and his colleagues argue that errors in areas which are specifically linguistic must be approached within a linguistic framework. LARSP provides such a framework. Furthermore, it provides a *systematic* means of planning remediation for these children.

That is not to say that LARSP cannot be used for working on the syntactic problems of children other than those with independent language difficulties. Here too, its precise detail and developmental orientation give an indication of the structural areas in which a child has difficulty and provides the starting point for remediation. This is exemplified in Crystal *et al.* (1976, pp. 113-17) where the more common profiles are described and related to remedial goals, the main aim being to bring the child down the LARSP chart 'in as controlled a way as possible' (p. 126).

This control is facilitated by the systematic nature of the chart, but at the same time, allows the clinician to decide on the techniques whereby the various structures are introduced and consolidated. LARSP also enables one to measure the efficacy of remedial methods by noting, for example, an increase in the number of structures previously used infrequently, and/or the use of new structures, and/or a progression to later stages.

Related Research

Part 2 of *Working with LARSP* (Crystal, 1979) is a compilation of reports by teachers and therapists experimenting with LARSP in various clinical settings. The contributors illustrate the usefulness of LARSP for planning remediation programmes which utilise such varied techniques as colour coding or signing. They also report that LARSP:

(i) is thorough, which helps in presenting carefully structured language which, in turn, develops the child's capacity for self-correction;

(ii) pinpoints specific persisting defects;
(iii) provides a systematic basis for building up a range of structures in a balanced way.

In this part, Auckland suggests that, given the hierarchical development of syntax, it would be useful to be able to pinpoint key relationships, i.e. those structures fundamental to development of later constructions, thereby making for 'easier recognition of . . . specific forms of remediation' (p. 212).

Brinton (1979) assesses the relationship between subjects' ability to imitate test sentences and their spontaneous language ability, as measured by LARSP. The correspondence which she found between expressive language and repetition tasks for linguistically normal children did not exist for the language delayed. This has implications for remediation in that it brings into question the usefulness of repetitive drills as a means of developing the syntax of the language delayed child.

Appraisal

Some of those having to deal with language problems may find this analysis rather daunting. Dever (1977), for instance, feels that it is too complex and lengthy for teachers faced with groups of children. He suggests that if Crystal *et al.* had followed through their assumption that certain grammatical patterns must be learned before others can be learned, the LARSP system could be rebuilt to allow the teacher to 'zero in' rapidly on the structures needing attention first. This proposal is similar to that of Auckland (1979).

Although the LARSP method of analysis is time-consuming and demanding, there are 'rewards' for the time taken, in that children for whom the test is suitable benefit from the detailed type of syntactic remediation plan derivable from LARSP.

Such a detailed representation of a child's abilities or disabilities, in a standard format, makes for easier comparison of profiles. These comparisons enable an appreciation of different patterns or areas of disability so that, with time, each can be related to the most effective method of treating it.

The lay-out of the Profile Chart clearly shows the gaps in the child's syntactic ability which provides a ready-made list of therapeutic goals. The Chart has, however, been criticised for the limited amount of information available at Stage I, but this section has been updated (Crystal, 1979) by means of a micro-profile which gives suggestions for assessment and remediation of children at or just below Stage I. Perera

(1980) considers this to be particularly useful for those working with the severely retarded.

The micro-profile also meets a criticism regarding the limitations of LARSP for dealing with syntactic comprehension problems. Hill and Wallace (1976, p. 156) suggest that the framework of LARSP 'is not ideally equipped to handle the various semantic and psycholinguistic factors which enter into comprehension difficulty'. The micro-profile provides further detail of the development of comprehension at Stage I and relates it to earlier perceptual development. Nevertheless, it is important to bear in mind that the authors do not claim a 'neat relationship' between comprehension and production, LARSP being designed primarily as a basis for work on the latter.

Developmental Sentence Analysis (DSA)

Theoretical Background

The purpose in designing this analysis (Lee, 1974) was to provide a detailed, part-scored evaluation of aspects of a child's language production, namely the use of grammatical rules. It is not a psycholinguistic study, though Lee admits that in formulating this technique for use by clinicians she has relied on insights gleaned from psycholinguistic research methods and findings.

Nor is DSA concerned with differential diagnostic procedures and classification of language pathologies. Rather it derives from the theory that a descriptive analysis based on normal development of grammatical structure assesses the child's incorporation of adult grammatical rules into spontaneous speech and, as such, is applicable to any clinical population.

The issue central to the division of this analysis into two sections (see 'Description') is Lee's concern with the child's adoption of subject-verb as the basic form of utterance. Thus, pre-sentences (containing partial subject-verb structure) are distinguished from complete sentences (where both subject and verb are spoken) and are evaluated separately as follows:

(i) pre-sentences on a Developmental Sentence Types (DST) chart;
(ii) complete sentences on a Developmental Sentence Scoring (DSS) sheet.

It is necessary at this stage to explain briefly the rationale underlying the classification of the DST into horizontal levels and vertical columns.

The latter arise from the need to distinguish between different kinds of sentences with different semantic contents or information while the horizontal levels are determined by the importance of increasing length of utterance in early language development (see 'Description' for detail).

The DSS, like the DST, also categorises the data, the reason for the selection of its eight categories of grammatical forms being that these show 'the most significant developmental progression' (p. 136) in children's language. Lee employs the terms of traditional grammar wherever possible as they are thought to be the most familiar to clinicians.

Description and Administration

Data are obtained from a tape-recorded sample of a child's spontaneous speech in conversation with an adult. From a transcription of the tape the assessor selects either 100 utterances for analysis by DST or 50 sentences by DSS. The following are suggested as guidelines when deciding on the procedure to employ:

(i) if corpus contains largely incomplete utterances, use DST;
(ii) if corpus contains 50 per cent/more complete sentences, use DSS; and
(iii) if more complete analysis required, use DST and DSS.

Of course, the continuous stream of speech produced by young children can create problems for the assessor attempting to structure the corpus of data in terms of separate utterances/sentences. Therefore, Lee (Chapter II) outlines certain rules which aid in this structuring.

Developmental Sentence Types. The chart is organised horizontally into three 'bands' or levels:

(i) single words;
(ii) two-word combinations;
(iii) multi-word constructions.

These levels combine with five vertical columns to form a fifteen-box grid, the vertical classification being:

(i) noun;
(ii) designator;
(iii) descriptive item;
(iv) verb;

(v) vocabulary item.

Lee gives many examples of the types of utterances appropriate to each box:

Table 2.3

	Designator-elaborated
Two-word combination	For example, designator + noun 'Here car'

	Verb-elaborated
Multi-word construction	For example, verb + object 'Eat the cookie'

When the child's utterances are entered into the chart the assessor is provided with a visual representation of that child's production patterns. In addition, the numbers of utterances at each level or in each column can be counted and compared with the language sample of 40 normally developing children by 3 month age groups (2.0 to 2.11 years) with regard to the mean number and standard deviations at each DST level and the percentage of utterances in each of the five DST sentence types. This enumeration is not, however, intended as a score.

Developmental Sentence Scoring. The eight grammatical categories for this section are:

(i) indefinite pronouns or noun modifiers;
(ii) personal pronouns;
(iii) main verbs;
(iv) secondary verbs;
(v) negatives;
(vi) conjunctions;
(vii) interrogative reversals;
(viii) Wh-questions.

Within each category progressively higher scores (ranging from 1 to 8) are given to structures which are supposedly later to develop in children's language learning, for example, personal pronouns, score 1 for 'I/me/you'; 3 for 'we/us'; and 7 for 'one/whatever'.

When all 50 sentences have been individually scored for these grammatical forms, the mean sentence score (DSS) is derived by totalling all the sentence scores and dividing by 50. A child's DSS can then be compared with that of normally developing children of the same chronological age by plotting the position of the score on the DSS norm chart. Children falling below the 10th percentile would warrant language intervention. The norms were derived from speech samples of 200 children, 5 girls and 5 boys at each 3-month age interval between the ages 2.0 and 6.11.

Therapeutic Implications

As DSA is constructed upon developmental stages of language acquisition it is useful for pinpointing the level of ability of the language delayed child thus indicating both the starting-point for and continuation of remediation. Where a general sense of language delay is complicated by total gaps in structural ability, the detailed information on normal grammatical development (Lee, 1974, Chapter I) provides a framework for concentration on specific areas of weakness.

Not only does such an analysis establish whether the child is following a normal pattern of grammatical development, it also indicates a possible irregular, atypical sequence of learning, in which case the child is far less likely to benefit from a remediation programme based on developmental progressions.

While DSA provides a systematic plan for presentation of syntactic structure in graded steps, it does not insist on a rigid adherence. Later structures can be introduced while continuing work on the expansion of earlier forms.

Using what she terms a 'clinical child' (language delayed, C.A. 3.7) as illustration, Lee describes useful goals of remediation. The orientation of DSA enables her to approach these on two levels; immediate goals, for example working on basic SVO formulation, verb elaboration and/or articles, and secondary goals, for example introducing plurals, personal pronouns and/or conjunctions.

Although the nature of these goals is essentially grammatical, Lee admits that remediation must go deeper than a concern merely for the surface form of utterances. She claims that children will not spontaneously use structures unless they recognise the relations that underlie them. With this in mind, she compares her own work with that of Brown (1973) on the development of (possibly universal) semantic relations in young children, and discovers striking parallels. This is significant for remediation as it points to the need for relating the two levels, for developing an awareness of semantic relations while teaching the grammatical forms which mark them.

Related Research

While studying mother-child verbal interaction, Rondal (1978) compared the conversational speech of 14 normal children with 14 Down's Syndrome children, using the DSS procedure for her analysis. She discovered that the Down's Syndrome group produced utterances which were syntactically less sophisticated, such as in the sequential ordering of main and secondary verbs. Rondal concluded her discussion with a plea for further such investigations which will allow 'a more precise tailoring of . . . language training and remedial programs to the specific needs of mentally retarded children' (p. 170).

Precision was also the concern of Daly (1978) who felt that elicited imitation was a procedure which could be effective in increasing the precision of assessment and clinical programming of children with language disorders. He cited a study by Cornelius (1974) which compared a group of language disordered and normal speaking children on Lee's DSS and Carrow's Elicited Imitation Inventory (1974). Cornelius found a statistically significant correlation between the two methods of collecting grammatical data. The implication of this finding, according to Daly, was that analysis of discrepancies between model and response pinpointed difficulties in children's 'productive rule capacities'. He suggested that elicited imitation was therefore as efficient and uncomplicated as DSS type procedure in obtaining information which was indicative of a child's remedial needs.

To continue with the issue of data collection as a basis for remediation (Lee recommends 50 sentences as appropriate for a speech sample),

Johnson and Tomblin (1975) considered that more than 50 sentences should be collected before DSS could be said to be reliable.

Appraisal

It could be argued that Lee's distinction between pre-sentence and sentence is adult-oriented. In relation to language acquisition such a rigid classification can be both difficult and misleading for there are 'functional and formal parallels' (Crystal *et al.*, 1976, p. 198) between pairs of utterances such as 'where car?' (DST) and 'where's car?' (DSS). Lee's justification of a separate DST class is that she is concerned with the final form of an utterance rather than with the possible semantic functions which may/may not be fully represented in the spoken form. Thus she chooses to ignore the common semantic intentions shared by the types of utterances exemplified above.

With regard to the DST, it does provide a systematic means of studying 'early' utterances, this being an area so often ignored in assessments. It also provides a means of judging a child's response to remediation; a downward flow on the chart indicates a progression of abilities. There is, however, a danger of merely counting the number of utterances at each DST level which does not show the qualitative differences between linguistically normal and abnormal children.

Another criticism by Crystal *et al.*(1976) is that Lee underestimates elliptical constructions by classifying them as incomplete. She upholds this classification on the grounds that frequent ellipsis points to a child who relies on deep structures formulated by the assessor, and/or does not initiate conversation.

The dependence of DSA on spontaneous language sampling may be a limitation for there are specific structures that are not often spontaneously produced by children (see Mulac, Prutting and Tomlinson, 1978). Further restrictions are imposed by Lee's choice of only eight grammatical categories on the DSS. However, in view of the need to keep the analysis as short as possible, these restrictions are understandable.

Test for Auditory Comprehension of Language* (TACL)

Theoretical Background

This test of Carrow's (1973) differs from Reynell's Verbal Comprehension Scale (1977) in that it is not formulated within a theory of con-

* Spanish and English versions have been designed but only the latter is discussed here.

ceptual development. It is concerned purely with early stages of a child's comprehension of the *structural* aspects of language. With regard to these aspects, Carrow argues that it is not sufficient to test comprehension merely at a vocabulary level, 'more complex' aspects must be included as these are the ones which so often present difficulty to those with comprehension problems.

TACL is a test designed to assign a child to a developmental level of comprehension. It is also intended to fulfil a diagnostic function by enabling the assessor to pinpoint the area(s) of linguistic difficulty. This is facilitated by the inclusion of an analysis section on the response form which allows for the grouping of items according to linguistic categories.

Most of the actual words used in this test are those which appear early in language acquisition. The inclusion of these words (for example, 'bicycle') as separate items at the beginning of the test is based on the theory that if the child has knowledge of them, any subsequent failure on the test may be safely attributed to difficulty with the grammatical form (for example, 'bicyclist' – derivational suffix) rather than with the lexical item itself.

Carrow claims that TACL is developmental, an increase in chronological age being reflected in an increasing score, but it is not developmental in the sense that test items are sequenced according to level of difficulty. The items are selected according to whether they assess knowledge of specific grammatical structures. This selection, determined by 'agreement of experts', is not concerned with the ability of the test items to discriminate between age groups.

Description and Administration

On this untimed test of 101 items only a picture pointing response is expected of the child. Of the pictures, three to a plate, one illustrates the linguistic form being tested and the others represent the contrasting forms. If, however, there is only one contrasting form, the third picture functions as a decoy.

As the test items are generally sequenced by grammatical category rather than by level of difficulty, the entire test must be administered. The structures tested are wide-ranging and, for the sake of clarity, are listed below according to the categories designated on the analysis section of the revised response sheet:

Vocabulary – nouns, adjectives, verbs and adverbs;
Morphology – suffixes, 'er', 'est', 'ist' + noun and/or verb and/or

adjective;
- number (nouns, pronouns and verbs);
- gender (pronouns);
- tense, voice and status (verbs);
- prepositions;
- interrogatives;

Syntax
- imperative;
- predication;
- modification;
- complementation.

Each correct pointing response is allotted one point, the total yielding the raw score which may then be converted to an age score. Conversion tables also provide the mean for age, standard deviations from the mean and a percentile rank.

Additional information is given on the response sheet in the form of age levels at which 75 per cent and 90 per cent of children pass *each* item. Also, as stated previously, there is provision for more detailed study (and structure subscores) on the analysis section which classifies more clearly the structure types included on the test.

The items on the revised response form referred to above are assigned to three subgroups (lexical, morphological and syntactic) while the norms in the manual show four subgroups, resulting from the separate listing of morphological construction and grammatical categories. Blood and Greenberg (1978) argue that this renders the norms inappropriate. They therefore established new norms for the revised test form.

Therapeutic Implications

As TACL incorporates more than the understanding of vocabulary, it goes someway to providing a means for identifying and guiding the remediation of general language comprehension problems. Its section on analysis of structure pinpoints more specific problems of comprehension thereby enabling more precise tailoring of a therapeutic programme to the child's needs. (But note the work by Millen and Prutting (1979) reviewed in the following section.)

The absence of a developmental orientation according to increasing levels of difficulty hinders the organisation of an orderly and sequential approach to remediation. Carrow assumes that the expression of grammatical patterns emerges in the same order as the understanding of them, which suggests that information on developmental order of forms in expressive language will provide guidelines for working on comprehension of these same forms. Not only is this neat parallelism unproven but also one has then to refer to sources other than TACL for the required information. Admittedly the author includes in the manual some references to work on comprehension but these are superficial and brief and do not provide any real guidance for designing a therapeutic programme.

This programme is further restricted because only a limited number of items are included for some structures, for example, adjective + derivational suffix 'est' – 1 item; direct-indirect object – 1 item. Also, the types of structures assessed are not representative of colloquial discourse. Although these restrictions also affect a clinician's assessment of the effectiveness of the remediation programme, it can still be said that TACL provides a broad framework for the planning of work on comprehension, the subgroups providing some means for evaluating improvement in performance in specific areas, as demonstrated by Weiner in 1972.

Related Research

Millen and Prutting's (1979) study attempted to determine if children responded differently across three tests of comprehension, one of which was TACL, the others being the Northwestern Syntax Screening Test: Receptive (Lee, 1969) and the Bellugi-Klima Comprehension Test (1971).

The thirteen children used as subjects were between the ages of 3.2 and 4.1. Comparison of their performances across tests showed significant differences for 11 of the 22 grammatical features under consideration. Although the Northwestern and TACL demonstrated consistent measurement on overall language comprehension scores, there were inconsistencies between the three tests with regard to *specific* features. The authors therefore concluded that the use of these test results to determine specific remediation goals 'would not appear clinically sound' (p. 169).

Determining test reliability was the basis to Anderson, Hess and Richardson's (1980) work on TACL. They studied 44 mentally retarded children, using a test-retest paradigm. Of the several results, those of interest were the facts that internal stability was highest for total score and that low co-efficients were obtained for the subtests of morphological construction and syntactic structure.

Thus Anderson *et al.* suggested that when these two subtests were considered independently, their value in assessing certain linguistic categories was questionable. As the subtests attempted to measure functions which were particularly immature in the retarded population they were probably inappropriate. The implication was that they would therefore be inadequate as a basis for detailed planning of remediation.

With regard to measuring improvement after remediation, the authors felt that subtest data alone were possibly not suitable for determining development of morphological construction and syntactic structure.

Appraisal

(See also comments under 'Therapeutic Implications'.)

While TACL distinguishes between children who have disorders of language comprehension and those who do not, its value as a basis for the planning of specific remediation is questionable. It seems to pinpoint comprehension problems in certain areas but whether these are truly representative of a child's disabilities has yet to be proven. It is certainly restricted in that only single, declarative sentences are used and, as pointed out by Rees and Shulman (1978), these are 'unrelated to one another or to any context other than the pictures presented for verification' (p. 209).

Furthermore, these pictures (all line drawings) do not always clearly represent the stimuli. Also they are more abstract than tasks involving three-dimensional objects.

The larger number of items on the test make it a time-consuming one to administer. However, in view of the earlier criticism regarding the limited number of types per token, it is difficult to envisage how a more comprehensive test could be designed which did not entail increased length. Perhaps more interesting illustrations would offset some of the potential boredom.

TACL is an American test but is suitable for British children as it includes very few Americanised words.

Despite the criticisms above, it must be said that Carrow attempts a linguistic categorisation of comprehension which is more precise and less vocabulary-oriented than many others. In fact, Blood and Greenberg (1978) consider TACL to be 'one of the most comprehensive measures of receptive language' (p. 210).

Conclusion

In this chapter, methods of analysing communication problems from a linguistic viewpoint have been described, concentrating on the phonological and grammatical aspects. While two of the assessments are termed tests of 'articulation' and supply largely phonetic information, they are included because they provide some insights into a child's patterning of sounds. Such information helps to clarify the way in which the child organises his language at a phonological level.

These tests have been selected to represent the range available to the clinician though attempts have been made to highlight the positive aspects of the measures whenever possible while maintaining an objective overall view of their usefulness for remediation. The section on therapeutic implications, related research and appraisal are particularly concerned with remedial issues. With regard to these issues, it will have been noted that the tests and techniques described vary in their suitability as bases for determining remediation in the areas they purport to assess.

These linguistic approaches are not seen as the panacea for assessment and remediation of language disorders. They are just a few of the methods available which can combine with methods from other fields of study in order to provide a comprehensive picture of a child's abilities and disabilities.

3 DEVELOPMENTAL PSYCHOLINGUISTIC APPROACHES

Chapter Outline

The importance of specific cognitive abilities for the development of language skills is discussed. It is argued that in remediating language, therapy should sometimes be directed towards improving specific cognitive abilities. Three tests for identifying psycholinguistic abilities are reviewed: the Reynell Developmental Language Scales, the Illinois Test of Psycholinguistic Abilities and the Aston Index. For each test, consideration is given to the theoretical background, to assessment, to therapeutic strategies and to related research, and an appraisal is made of each. It is suggested that both the Reynell and the Aston are particularly useful for 'screening' purposes and that the value of the ITPA lies in its diagnostic approach. However, it is pointed out that it might be time to undertake a revision of the subtests included in the ITPA in the light of recent research.

Introduction

Developmental psycholinguistics emphasises the relationship between cognitive abilities and language performance. This approach is based on the notion that language depends upon, and is connected with, a number of specific cognitive abilities, including memory, auditory and visual perception, symbolic understanding, categorising, discriminating and sequencing. It is these conceptual processes that are seen as helping children develop the skills of language.

This analysis of the relationship between cognition and language implies that in the remediation of deficient language performance, therapy should be directed towards improving specific cognitive abilities. Similarly, many American researchers have adopted the 'learning disabilities' approach in which children are seen as having specific learning disabilities which affect school performance and hinder social and cognitive growth. In many cases these children have been found to have average IQ's and their problem is attributed to inadequate learning strategies. An interesting discussion of the educational problems arising from learning disabilities can be found in Farnham-

Diggory (1978).

Stott (1978) has put forward the interesting argument that for children with learning disabilities it is better to think in terms of the non-use or poor use of capabilities, rather than of deficits. He suggests that remediation should be directed towards exercising these abilities and that children need encouragement to use previously under-used skills. This he argues depends upon helping children become motivated to cope with their environment and to learn effectively.

Whether these abilities are deficient or simply under-used is an important question. The first step in finding the answer, is the precise assessment of those cognitive skills which are related to language, bearing in mind the importance of attempting to make a diagnosis, as discussed in Chapter 1. Three tests for identifying psycholinguistic abilities will be examined and their usefulness in assessing and remediating deficient language performance discussed.

The Reynell Developmental Language Scales

Theoretical Background

The revised edition of the Reynell Developmental Language Scales (RDLS) is probably the test used most widely by speech therapists, particularly in Britain, to assess children's language. It consists of two separate scales which assess verbal comprehension and verbal expression independently. The original experimental version of the test covered the age range 6 months to 6 years and was designed to be most sensitive over the age range 1½ to 4 years. In constructing the revised edition, special emphasis was given to increasing the sensitivity of the test for children up to 6 years. At the same time the spread of items at the beginning of the verbal comprehension scale was increased and the scoring and instructions for the expressive scale were altered to help elicit as much language as possible from shy children. An attempt was also made to make the scales more suitable for hearing impaired children.

The theoretical background of the RDLS has been described in detail by Reynell (1969; 1972; 1976) and will only be referred to briefly. Her view of language development appears to have been heavily influenced by the work of Vygotsky (1962) and Luria (1961). Figure 3.1 illustrates Reynell's model of the integration of some of the processes involved in the development of verbal language. This suggests that at around the age of 5 years language becomes internalised as a vehicle to direct and regulate behaviour, as suggested by Luria.

Figure 3.1: Language Development

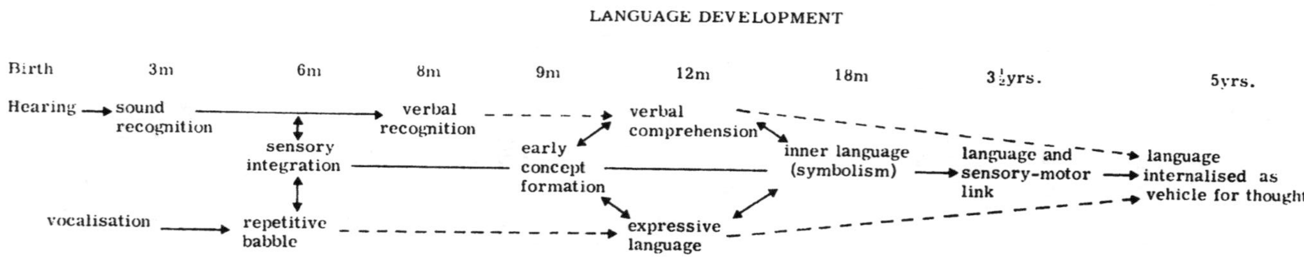

Source: From Reynell, 1969. Reproduced by special permission from the author and the *British Journal of Disorders of Communication.*

The implications of this model for assessing language development are illustrated in Figure 3.2. It can be seen that at each age range verbal comprehension and expressive language are paralleled by the development of cognitive abilities, referred to by Reynell as 'symbolic understanding'. These suggested links demonstrate ways in which cognitive activities and language performance may be related.

Description and Administration

Reynell's approach to assessment is derived directly from her model of language development as can be seen from Figure 3.3. Each of these aspects is assessed separately in order to identify areas in which children may be in need of specialised therapeutic help. The overall emphasis of the RDLS is on assessing concept formation and symbolic understanding which are included in both the verbal comprehension and expressive language components.

These scales are described fully in the manual for the revised edition (Reynell, 1977). The Verbal Comprehension Scale 'A' includes a range of tasks, from quite simple activities such as relating one symbol (a word) to another symbol (a toy), to more complex activities such as putting 'all the white pigs round the outside of the field' (p. 16). Intermediate tasks include relating two objects, such as putting a spoon in a cup and at a slightly higher level relating attributes such as colour, size and position.

There is also a Verbal Comprehension Scale 'B' for use with children who have no speech and poor motor control. Reynell suggests that this scale is useful for children who are very shy. Scale 'B' follows the same developmental sequence as Scale 'A'.

The Expressive Language Scale is divided into three Sections which loosely follow a developmental pattern and at the same time allow some overlap. Section 1 is concerned with the structure of language and assesses spontaneous expression. The first part of Section 1 covers simple vocalisation, including single-syllable sounds and double syllable babble, until children are able to use definite words referring to verbal concepts. The remainder of this Section assesses the ability to combine words, produce simple sentences and use complex sentences. Section 2 assesses vocabulary using objects, pictures and finally words alone. Initially children are asked to respond to questions of the form 'what is this?' but eventually have to define the meaning of words such as 'sleeping'. In Section 3 an attempt is made to assess the creative use of language through describing pictures. Credit is given for simply describing a set picture, but more importantly for linking ideas in sentences

Figure 3.2: Approximate Ages at which some of the Stages of Language Development are Acquired

Approximate age	Symbolic understanding (non-verbal language)	Verbal comprehension	Expressive verbal language
8–10 months	Early concept formation Awareness of permanence of objects	Some situational understanding of phrase patterns	Patterned vocalisation
12 months	Object recognition	Appropriate response to familiar phrases	Expressive jargon
15–18 months	Early symbolic recognition Large doll-play	A few verbal labels understood	Uses a few recognisable words
18–21 months	Basic symbolic understanding established Small doll-play Recognises clear coloured pictures	Selects familiar objects in response to naming	Vocabulary of 12+ words
2–2½ years	Relates symbol to symbol Matches toys to pictures	Relates two named objects 'put the *spoon* in the *cup*'	Names familiar objects Word combinations
2½–3 years	Understands more arbitrary symbols Relates gesture to picture	Selects object by use 'which do we cook with?'	Uses short sentences including prepositions and pronouns
3–4 years		Follows increasingly complex verbal directions containing 3 to 4 'operative' words per sentence	Fluent sentences – usually of mature structure by 4 years

Source: From Reynell, 1976, pp. 130-1. Reproduced by special permission from *Language and Communication in General Practice* edited by B. Tanner. Copyright 1976. Published by Hodder and Stoughton Educational.

and for producing additional sentences of relevance to the picture. Clearly, Sections 1 and 3 rely considerably on the ability of the tester to observe accurately and interpret children's vocalisations.

Figure 3.3: Processes Involved in Language Development Relating to Assessment

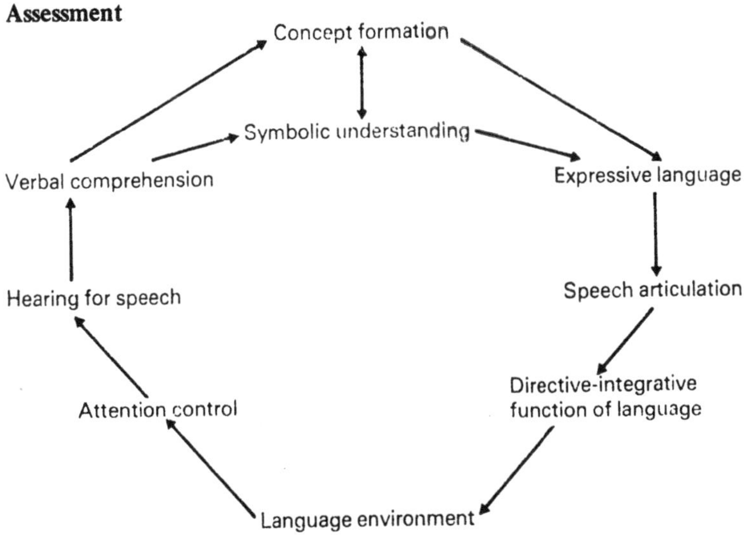

Source: From Reynell, 1976, p. 119. Reproduced by special permission from *Language and Communication in General Practice* edited by B. Tanner. Copyright 1976. Published by Hodder and Stoughton Educational.

The Scales have been primarily standardised on children from London and the South East of England with the inclusion of a small sample from the North of England. Selection of the children was based entirely on age although those whose mother tongue was not English were omitted. The total sample of children was 1318 (662 boys and 656 girls). Reynell (1977) herself notes, that care should be exercised in using the Scales in areas of Great Britain where standardisation has not taken place and that variables such as social class which have not been included in the standardisation should be taken into account when interpreting test scores. However, the Scales are designed to be widely used in assessing the expressive and comprehension abilities of children in Great Britain.

As pointed out the main feature of the test is that it has separate Scales to measure different aspects of language performance. This enables any obvious differences between children's understanding of language and their ability to communicate through the use of language to be identified. Implicit in Reynell's model is that comprehension precedes production and that therapy should be planned accordingly. However, as pointed out by Bloom and Lahey (1978, Chapter VIII), this may not always be the case. Although this form of assessment does indicate to the therapist possible approaches to remediation, it must be noted that for there to be statistically significant differences between the Scales, the difference between the standard scores needs to be approximately two standard deviations. This very large difference limits the sensitivity of the test in any comparison of the two Scales and should be held in mind by those planning therapy.

The Scales have formed the basis for a developmental programme for children with early language handicaps (Cooper, Moodley and Reynell, 1978). The procedures were devised and developed in the Wolfson Centre at the Institute of Child Health, London, and provide a comprehensive guide to assessing children's language performance in relationship to cognitive, social and physical factors. To accomplish this, it is suggested that all children presenting with language difficulties should have a paediatric assessment and hearing tests prior to treatment.

Cooper *et al.* (1978) argue that psychological assessment needs to be broken down into different aspects of intellectual functioning in order to identify the level and pattern of learning that individual children might be using. It is suggested that the following abilities should be assessed: attention control; symbolic understanding; concept formation; non-linguistic performance; verbal comprehension; expressive language; and the intellectual use of language. These are very similar to the areas shown in Reynell's model in Figure 3.3.

Attention control is assessed on the basis of children's responses to any tasks requiring their involvement, and follows the schedule shown in Figure 3.4. It is suggested that symbolic understanding be assessed by the Symbolic Play Test (Lowe and Costello, 1976) or through a series of matching activities (see Cooper *et al.*, 1978, pp. 39-41). They have also devised a schedule for assessing concept formation, which includes the understanding of in, out, left, right, and so forth. Included in non-linguistic performance are tasks of visual perception such as matching shapes, and a variety of constructional tasks. Verbal comprehension and expressive language are assessed on the basis of the RDLS, and the intellectual use of language is assessed through observation during tests and during free play.

This battery of tests is particularly useful prior to planning therapy. Cooper *et al.* (1978) provide a number of assessment schedules which are easy to administer and help build up a comprehensive picture of any individual child's ability. They also enable progress to be carefully monitored. Combined with the RDLS the schedule developed by Cooper *et al.* (1978) would seem to have a number of therapeutic implications for therapists, teachers and psychologists concerned with language development.

Figure 3.4: Attention Schedule

NAME:

D.O.B.: DATE:

ATTENTION CONTROL												
1. CAN PAY FLEETING ATTENTION THOUGH HIGHLY DISTRACTIBLE												
2. RIGID ATTENTION TO OWN CHOICE OF ACTIVITY												
3. SINGLE CHANNEL ATTENTION: CAN ATTEND TO ADULT'S CHOICE OF ACTIVITY—BUT UNDER ADULT CONTROL												
4. SINGLE CHANNEL ATTENTION: UNDER CHILD'S OWN CONTROL												
5. INTEGRATED ATTENTION: FOR SHORT SPELLS												
6. INTEGRATED ATTENTION: WELL CONTROLLED AND SUSTAINED												

CODE: GRADES	COMMENTS:
1. OCCASIONALLY 2. MOST OF THE TIME BUT FLUCTUATING 3. STABLE	

Source: Reproduced by special permission from *Helping Language Development. A Developmental Programme for Children with Early Language Handicaps* by J. Cooper, M. Moodley and J. Reynell. Copyright 1978. Published by Edward Arnold.

Therapeutic Implications

Comprehensive guidelines for therapy are provided by Cooper *et al.* (1978, Chapter 4) and these formed the basis for the Wolfson Language Developmental Programme described above. In their book, detailed information is provided on how to foster development in those areas in which assessment has taken place. The following suggestions are based on their ideas.

Work on attention control is considered to be very important. Initial emphasis is placed on helping children focus their attention on anything that is intrinsically interesting to them. Next they are encouraged to undertake activities free from any direct interference from therapists or teachers who might be working on the same task themselves, whilst indirectly providing a verbal commentary. Children are then taught how to adapt to adult initiated directions by gaining extrinsic reinforcement (material rewards), which are eventually replaced by the activity becoming socially reinforcing in itself. This then becomes internalised so that children can respond to directions from adults without direct teaching. Finally, children are taught how to deal with two tasks simultaneously.

The fostering of visual perception and visuo-motor abilities is undertaken primarily by initiating play activities at the appropriate developmental level of the child. Hence, it is suggested that early work on visual perception include shape matching and jigsaw puzzles. Later at a more advanced stage, children are encouraged to use language to help them describe pictures which differ slightly in content. Similarly, visuomotor abilities may be facilitated by helping children to copy three dimensional models and be concluded by encouraging them to create their own models. Again the therapist is encouraged to adopt an active role by making specific suggestions which correspond to the children's level of development.

The teaching programme for concept formation included in Cooper *et al.* (1978) follows predetermined stages. Colours are taught first followed by matching tasks involving the giving of verbal labels. Next classification skills are taught, which include sorting objects into categories according to colour, type, or shape. This leads on to sorting by use, for example, things used for eating. Then the concepts of size and quantities are taught until children are able to order more than two comparisons. Finally, positional concepts such as 'under', 'behind' and 'in front of' are introduced. There is a wealth of material available in this area to help therapists and teachers, but what is especially interesting about the Wolfson programme, is the suggested order of development.

The teaching of symbolic understanding follows a similar pattern. Through play activities, children are taught recognition of normal size objects followed by the same objects in a smaller symbolic form. They are then encouraged to undertake large doll play to foster imaginative activities which leads on to small doll play. This is followed by a series of matching activities including toys to pictures, pictures to toys, gestures to pictures, and pictures to gestures. Gestures are used together with the spoken word and not in isolation. The inclusion of gesture is interesting especially in the light of recent work by Lock (1978) on the relationship between the evolution of language and gesture.

Verbal comprehension, it is suggested by Cooper *et al.* (1978), is in the early stages very much more important than expressive language and consequently should be taught first. They make various suggestions for teaching different stages of verbal understanding. The pattern suggested is as follows: relating two named objects, e.g. 'put the spoon in the box'; relating nouns and verbs; relating nouns and adjectives; and finally, understanding long sentences. Expressive language is not taught directly until a firm basis for comprehension is established. Therapists and teachers are then encouraged to help expand utterances by providing sentences to be completed and by direct questioning. It should be noted that the implicit assumption in this approach to therapy, is that language is learned and hence can be taught through what might be termed behavioural strategies. This idea which has been reviewed by Müller (1980) will be discussed further in Chapter 6.

The overall aim of the programme as already mentioned, is to foster the use of language as a directive and integrative activity for further intellectual development. It is suggested that this aim should be considered at all times, and that children should be encouraged to use language to work out their problems and to monitor their own behaviour.

Related Research

Cooper, Moodley and Reynell (1974, 1979) have made careful attempts to monitor the effectiveness of the Wolfson programme. Their later paper is the most comprehensive review available and will be considered in some detail.

Cooper *et al.* (1979) implemented the 'Preschool Developmental Language Programme' both in 'languages classes' consisting of 8 children under the direction of a teacher, and in 'language clinics' by parents under the supervision of a speech therapist who they met every 6 weeks. The age range of the children was from 2 to 4½ years. Excluded were severely deaf children and those with severe physical handicaps. Quantitative assessments were made annually in the areas of attention control, symbolic understanding, concept formation, performance skills (non-verbal), verbal comprehension and expressive language. These were carried out on the basis of age equivalent scores and progress was rated as 'good', 'steady' or 'poor'.

They adopted an interesting methodology for rating progress. 'Steady' progress over a year was indicated by the equivalent of one year's progress for a child, plus or minus 3 months. Anything outside these limits was rated as 'good' or 'poor'. A year's progress however, was estimated according to the previous rate of development. Hence a 3 year old child presenting with a language age of 2 years, is assumed to have progressed at a rate of two-thirds his age. If this child were to improve over the year by two-thirds of a year plus 4 months, this would be considered as good progress.

This method of calculating progress is not without criticism, predicting as it does that if at the age of 3 a child is progressing at a rate of two-thirds his age, that the same mathematical formula will apply at a later age, such that at 6 years the child would have a language age of 4 years, at 9 years one of 6 years, and at 12 years one of 8 years. Furthermore, given the above example, the child's progress would be rated 'good' if at the age of 4 years his language age was 3 years or above (8 months plus 4 months). Many therapists and teachers might wish to query this.

The results of this study are shown in Figures 3.5 and 3.6. A large proportion of the children made considerable progress in both the language 'classes' and 'clinics'. In particular, verbal comprehension and verbal expression showed a marked rate of progress. This can be interpreted as showing the validity of a therapeutic programme directed at related cognitive abilities as well as at language itself. Follow-up studies after the children had completed the programme and had started school, demonstrated that the advantages gained had been maintained even though progress had been slowed down a little.

A further study was conducted to ascertain the programme's effectiveness. The progress of the children in the programme was compared with a group having no help and a group having conventional weekly speech therapy. The percentage of each sample making 'accelerated' progress in verbal comprehension and expressive language was recorded. Although those having conventional speech therapy appeared to have progressed more than those having no therapy, the most success was gained by those following the Wolfson programme. Cooper *et al.* (1979, p. 65) conclude that 'the procedures are valid in relation to the aims, and are adaptable to a number of different settings in both class and clinic'.

However, it must be pointed out that in some ways the experimental group had advantages over the control groups, one uncontrollable factor obviously being the time spent receiving therapy. The Wolfson programme provided daily help either from teachers or from using parents as teachers. Furthermore, it can legitimately be argued that the quantification of progress was not very precise. However, despite these comments, the research of Cooper *et al.* (1979) is a clear statement of the benefits which seem to accrue from the use of a structured language programme.

Figure 3.5: The Rate of Progress of the Language Class Children During Their Time in the Class for the Five Measurable Areas of Development

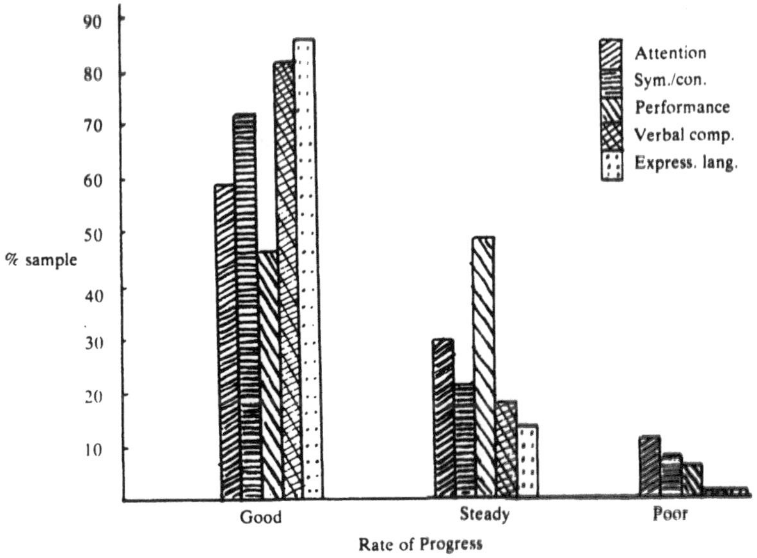

Source: From Cooper, Moodley and Reynell, 1979. Reproduced by special permission from the authors and the *British Journal of Disorders of Communication.*

Appraisal

Before appraising the usefulness of the Reynell Developmental Language Scales for planning therapy, it should be noted that therapeutic programmes based upon them are still at an experimental stage. The revised edition was only completed in 1977 and the results of the Wolfson project which incorporated a great deal of the theoretical background derived from Reynell's model, only became available in 1979. However, there are a number of points which should be made.

The theoretical model which Reynell puts forward is in many ways limited. It is no longer certain that comprehension precedes production, and work by Nelson (1973) for example, has shown how infants can learn the meaning of words through simply using them. Furthermore, the emphasis given to the internalisation of language to foster thinking rather limits the richness of children's cognitive activities which seem to prepare the way for language. MacNamara (1972) for example, argues strongly that the infant uses meaning as a clue to language, rather than language as a clue to meaning, and he further suggests that the infant adopts an active role in acquiring the prerequisite skills for communication. Similarly, the work on attention seems particularly naive in the light of far more sophisticated models of information processing, as for example put forward by Broadbent (1971).

Figure 3.6: The Rate of Progress for the Language Class Sample Between the Time of Admission to the Developmental Language Programme and the Final Follow Up after Leaving the Class

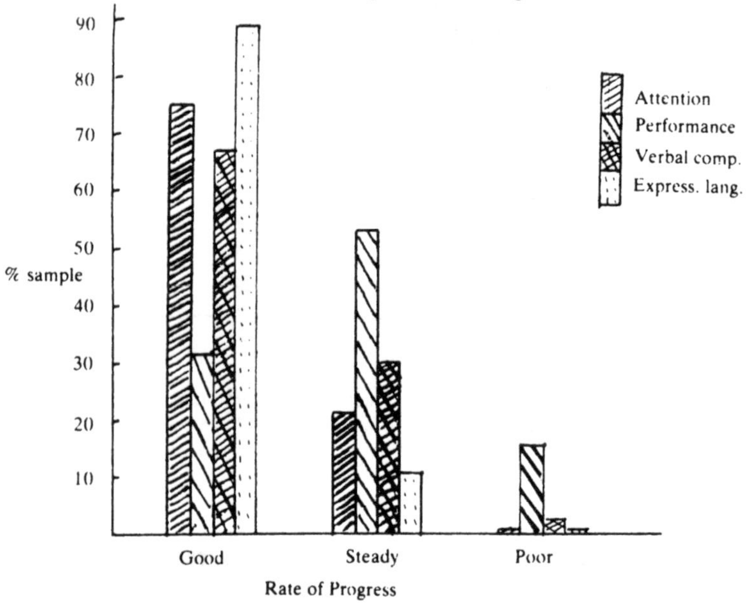

Source: From Cooper, Moodley and Reynell, 1979. Reproduced by special permission from the authors and the *British Journal of Disorders of Communication.*

Crystal *et al.* (1976) criticise the Expressive Scale for failing to incorporate specific linguistic structures into the assessment, unlike the LARSP which is based on a more exact syntactic description of language (see Chapter 2). Also, there is no clear rationale underlying the selection of those syntactic features which are included in the Expressive Scale. For instance, does the suggestion 'give credit for the number of complete sentences' refer to completeness of grammaticality or of conceptualisation? The ambiguity arises due to the fact that the instruction appears in the Content Section which is purported to assess 'creative' uses of language as opposed to language structure.

In interpreting the actual scores obtained from the Scales, further problems arise. It is uncertain if the Scales are diagnostic or whether in fact they simply describe the development of cognitive functions such as attention and concept formation. As in so many tests, this makes it difficult to measure improvement especially as therapy often revolves around the teaching of the test itself. Certainly, the Wolfson programme can be criticised on these grounds, although it can still be argued that this is a valid and legitimate therapeutic activity.

A second point on test interpretation, is that a very small range of raw scores covers quite a wide range of ability. For example, on the Expressive Scale only 6 points cover -3 to -2 standard deviations at the age of 4 years. This makes it possible for only small differences in the performance of 4 year old children to make quite a marked difference in their recorded ability. This is particularly important as the Scales seem to be used more often to assess children having difficulty with language, all of whom tend to have a restricted range of ability. Thus, where the test should be most accurate it may not in fact do much more than indicate a possible problem.

Set against this, is the success of the Wolfson project and the fact that the Reynell is the only readily available standardised test encompassing verbal comprehension and expression. Certainly, the evidence presented above does suggest that the Scales can be useful in guiding therapy and in this sense they can be seen as diagnostic. Furthermore, there may be nothing wrong in teaching test items if these enable improved language performance to generalise to other situations. In this way the Scales can be seen as criterion rather than norm referenced. This simply means that they may serve to set a standard for children to reach and in so doing give clear indications for therapy.

Given that the Scales can point to where therapy may be needed, it is reasonable to suggest that they might be most useful in screening children with suspected language problems. Certainly, Stevenson and Richman (1976) found a very simplified version of the Expressive Scale useful in identifying the prevalence of language delay in 3 year old children. In conclusion, it is apparent that the Scales are meeting a definite need, particularly for speech therapists, and research should be encouraged to evaluate the most appropriate and effective ways of using them.

The Illinois Test of Psycholinguistic Abilities

Theoretical Background

The experimental edition of the Illinois Test of Psycholinguistic Abilities (ITPA) was revised by Kirk, McCarthy and Kirk in 1968, and it is this version which is currently in use. Compared to the Reynell Developmental Language Scales, the ITPA assesses a wider variety of psycholinguistic abilities in order to identify those specific areas in which children might require remedial help. Single overall test scores were seen as being too broad to indicate possible therapy, and it was argued that by identifying and remediating specific deficient cognitive abilities, language and other related skills would also improve. In this sense, Kirk *et al.* claim that the ITPA is a diagnostic rather than a classificatory tool.

The ITPA was based on a model of the communication process first proposed by Osgood in the late fifties (Kirk *et al.*, 1968). An account of the development of the ITPA can be found in Paraskevopoulos and Kirk (1969) and will be described briefly in this chapter.

The model is three dimensional and distinguishes between: (a) channels of communication; (b) psycholinguistic processes; and (c) levels of organisation.

(a) **Channels of Communication.** These are routes through which the the content of communication flows. The major modes of input are auditory and visual, and output is usually either vocal or motor. The ITPA incorporates two main channels; auditory-vocal where information is received through the ear and the response is verbal, and visual-motor where information is received through the eye and the response is manual.

(b) **Psycholinguistic Processes.** Three main processes are identified as being involved in the acquisition and use of language. The *receptive process* is the ability to understand and/or recognise what is seen or heard, and is concerned with input. Vocal or sensori-motor output is controlled by the *expressive processes*. In between are the associative, or more precisely the *organising processes*, which involve the internal manipulation of percepts, concepts and linguistic symbols in order to mediate between input and output.

(c) **Levels of Organisation**. These refer to the degree to which 'habits of communication have been developed' (Paraskevopoulos and Kirk, 1969, p. 14). At the 'automatic' level the individual's habits of communication are highly organised and result in automatic chains of responses. The 'representational level' requires the internal manipulation and reorganisation of symbols and the process of communication is less automatic and more thoughtful.

Theoretically, this model indicates twelve possible areas for assessment (2 channels of communication x 3 psycholinguistic processes x 2 levels of organisation). In practice, more emphasis is given to the representational level where all six areas are assessed (2 channels of communication x 3 psycholinguistic processes). At the automatic level, emphasis is placed entirely on the organising processes involving both channels of communication and not on either receptive or expressive processes. The next section will describe these subtests in more detail.

Description and Administration

The ITPA consists of ten subtests and two supplementary tests. At the representational level there are six subtests as follows; two assessing the receptive process, two assessing the organising process and two the expressive process.

(a) **The Receptive Process**
(i) *Auditory Reception*. This test assesses the ability to understand simple sentences such as 'Do dogs eat?' or 'Do dials yawn?' The response throughout is kept at a simple yes/no level.
(ii) *Visual Reception*. In this test the child is shown one picture for 3 seconds and then presented with 4 response pictures on a second page from which the one that is 'like' the stimulus picture has to be selected. Only pointing is required.

(b) **The Organising Process**
(i) *Auditory Association*. This assesses the ability to complete verbal analogies of the type, 'Soup is hot, ice-cream is . . .'
(ii) *Visual Association*. This test requires the child to associate concepts presented visually by matching the stimulus with one of four pictures, e.g. sock with shoe, or hammer with nail.

(c) **The Expressive Process**
(i) *Verbal Expression*. In this test the child is shown simple objects

and asked to say as much as possible about them.

(ii) *Manual Expression.* This test requires the child to mime the appropriate action linked to pictures of common objects, e.g. a guitar or a telephone.

At the automatic level only the organising processes are assessed. Kirk *et al.* (1968) suggest that two general abilities are measured at this level, 'closure' and 'short term sequential memory'.

(a) **Closure**

(i) *Grammatic Closure.* This test requires the child to finish incomplete statements and assesses the ability to select the correct grammatical form corresponding to set pictures. For example, the examiner might say 'Here is a dog; here are two . . .'; or 'This dog likes to bark; here he is . . .'

(ii) *Visual Closure.* This test assesses the child's ability to identify common objects which are incomplete and partially hidden amongst others.

Evesham (1980) notes that, although the test of grammatic closure was placed on the automatic level, Kirk and Kirk (1978) now consider that it would be more correctly placed at the representational level with auditory and visual association. In addition the two supplementary tests also involve closure.

(iii) *Auditory Closure.* In this test the child has to complete a word by filling in the missing part, e.g. *bo / le* (bottle), *tele / one* (telephone).

(iv) *Sound Blending.* This is similar to auditory closure and requires the child to identify a word when individual parts are spoken at half-second intervals, e.g. *f-oot* or *d-i-nn-er*.

(b) **Sequential Memory**

(i) *Auditory Sequential Memory.* This requires the child to recall sequences of digits increasing from two to eight digits.

(ii) *Visual Sequential Memory.* In this test the child has to recall and reproduce sequences of non-meaningful figures.

Despite the fact that these subtests are designed to assess discrete psycholinguistic abilities, it is stressed that children have to integrate these functions. Paraskevopoulos and Kirk (1969) illustrate this by noting the processes involved in describing and interpreting a picture.

First, children must understand the instruction (auditory reception), and secondly, they have to understand the meaning of the picture (visual reception) which they then have to relate to past experiences (visual association). Finally, the picture and its meaning have to be explained verbally (verbal expression). The integration of these abilities into goal directed activities is similar to the developmental model put forward by Reynell (1969).

The ITPA has been standardised in the USA on a sample of approximately 1000 'average' children between the ages of 2 to 10. This sample was selected as being of average performance on 'traditional measures of intelligence, school achievement and socioeconomic status and of intact motor and sensory development' (Kirk *et al.*, 1968, p. 93). It should be noted that unlike the Reynell, this normative data is derived from pre-selected average children rather than from children selected purely on the basis of age. Marinosson (1974) has published performance profiles for matched normal, educationally subnormal and severely subnormal children in English schools which can be used to supplement the American norms. Mittler (1976) points out though, that the application of the ITPA to the severely educational subnormal is limited as it cannot yield useful results below a language age of 3½ to 4 years. Evesham (1980) also notes that it is more reliable with children aged between 4 and 8 years. However, in order to help standardise the administration and interpretation of the ITPA, Kirk (1974) has produced a very detailed guide for test users.

As already pointed out, the ITPA is an attempt to isolate and assess discrete cognitive abilities to enable remediation to be planned accordingly. The subtests provide three types of norms: a Composite Psycholinguistic Age, Psycholinguistic Age Norms and Scaled Scores for each of the subtests. Kirk *et al.* (1968) administered the Short Form of the Stanford-Binet Intelligence Scale and found a close correspondence between the Composite Psycholinguistic Age and Binet Mental Age (see Table D, page 226, Paraskevopoulos and Kirk, 1969). It is proposed that a child's psycholinguistic age can be used as a rough estimate of overall intellectual development. However, an overall score is of limited value in planning remediation and is only useful for classifying children at certain levels of development.

It is through the use of Psycholinguistic Age Norms and in particular Scaled Scores for each subtest, that specific therapeutic programmes can be planned. The age norms are useful as a means of indicating where specific problems may lie, but they can be a little deceptive. Kirk *et al.* (1968) note that it is difficult to make direct comparisons between subtests using age norms because each test has a different range of raw scores.

Instead, therapeutic planning should be derived from the Scaled Scores for each subtest. The Scaled Scores are raw scores transformed so that at each age and for all twelve subtests the mean performance is equal to a score of 36 with a standard deviation of 6. This means that in the case of the ITPA subtests, more than 80 per cent of average children score between 30 and 42. It is these Scaled Scores which are used to construct a Profile of Abilities.

To establish whether or not a child has discrepancies in abilities the overall performance is expressed in terms of either the Mean or Median Scaled Score. The Median Scaled Score is more appropriate with profiles in which extremely discrepant scores are either all high or low. By comparing the difference between the Scaled Score of a subtest and the Mean or Median Scaled Score, the degree of strength and weakness in specific functions can be identified.

Kirk *et al.* (1968) suggest the following guidelines:

(i) differences of between + and -6, should not be considered as an indication of a special ability or deficit;
(ii) differences of between + or -7, 8 and 9, are considered as borderline discrepancies;
(iii) differences greater than + or -10, indicate discrepant functioning in relationship to the child's overall ability.

For example, from the profile in Figure 3.7 it can be seen that this child has particular visual deficiencies as well as related difficulties with expression, both manually and verbally. In contrast, Figure 3.8 presents a profile of a mentally retarded child (Kirk and Kirk, 1971, p. 92) with no specific disabilities or strengths, who is equally affected in all his psycholinguistic abilities.

This last example indicates the importance of making a clinical judgement on all the information collected. First, global scores give an overall appraisal of how well the child is functioning. Secondly, the psycholinguistic age norms for each subtest may indicate possible areas for remediation and enable comparisons to be made with children of the same age. Finally, by using Scaled Scores it is possible to diagnose precisely those deficiencies relative to the child's overall level of functioning. If these are markedly discrepant, therapeutic techniques can be directed at these specific weaknesses.

Figure 3.7: Profile for Scaled Scores for a Mentally Retarded Child with no Substantial Abilities or Disabilities

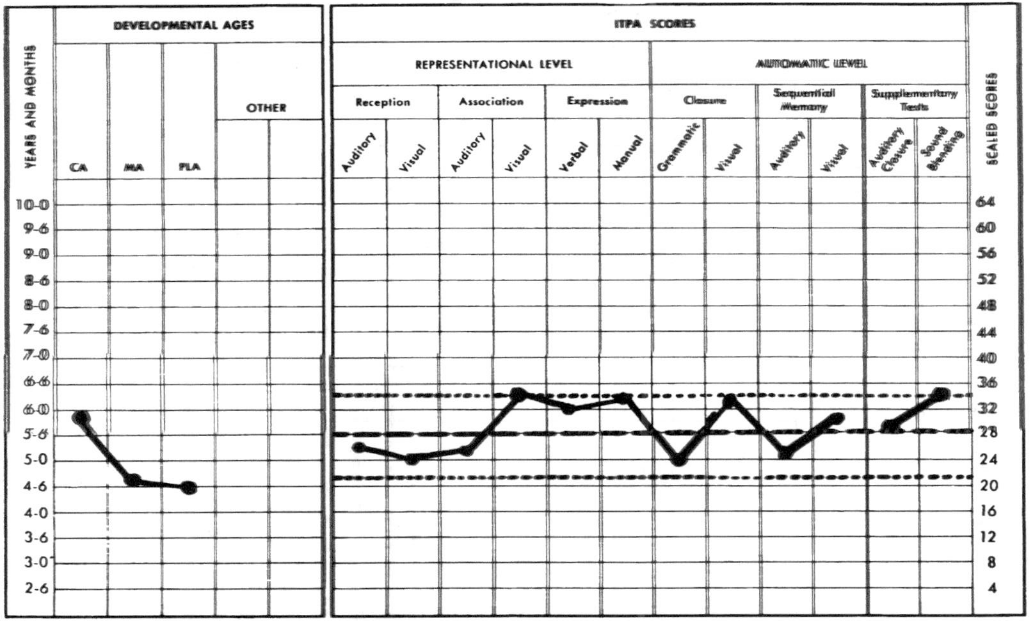

Source: Reproduced by special permission from *Psycholinguistic Learning Disabilities: Diagnosis and Remediation* by S.A. Kirk and W.D. Kirk. Copyright 1971. Published by the University of Illinois Press.

There has been considerable discussion in the literature about ways of determining statistically significant differences between subtest scores (Paraskevopoulos and Kirk, 1969; Kirk and Kirk, 1971; Lavine, 1978; Tierney and Ames, 1978). From a therapeutic viewpoint, it can be argued that this approach is misleading as it suggests that only statistically significant results are important (Müller, in press). Clearly, a child performing poorly on one or more subtests may benefit from therapy whether or not these discrepancies are statistically significant. A similar argument can be applied to differentiating between the Expressive and Comprehension Scales of the Reynell.

Figure 3.8: Profile of Scaled Scores for a Child with Visual and Expressive Difficulties

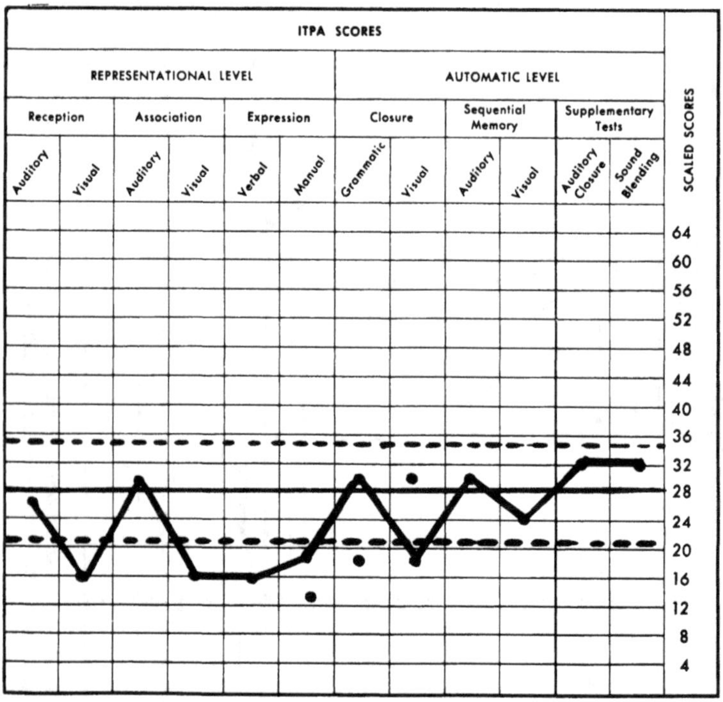

Source: Record Form reproduced by special permission from the *Illinois Test of Psycholinguistic Abilities* by S.A. Kirk, J.J. McCarthy and W.D. Kirk. Copyright 1968. Published by the University of Illinois Press.

Finally, mention should be made of a shortened version of the ITPA which has been developed by Newcomer and Hammill (1974), but as yet has not been standardised on a very large sample of children. Although designed as a screening test, Maggiore (1978) in examining the reliability of the shortened version, concluded that the 'user who encounters time difficulties should administer only the subtests of interest rather than reduce each subtest's length and as a consequence its reliability' (p. 204). However, this conclusion has in turn been disputed by Hammill and Newcomer (1980).

It is clear that the ITPA has been devised with therapy in mind and the vast amount of research on its use bears witness to this. The next two sections will examine some of the research which has derived therapeutic techniques from the test, and will evaluate the efficacy of this approach.

Therapeutic Implications

As compared to the Reynell Developmental Language Scales, there is a great deal of material available to help therapists work with the ITPA. One useful source is Kirk and Kirk (1971, Chapters 8 and 9). They suggest that teachers and therapists need to ascertain the levels, processes and channels towards which therapy should be directed. Kirk and Kirk (1971) suggest guidelines and suitable activities for remediating the main areas assessed. Rather than providing actual material in a structured programme, they indicate the kind of remedial approach needed and leave the therapist or the teacher to implement treatment.

In contrast, Karnes (1972) has devised an extremely structured language development programme based specifically on the ITPA. (The programme is entitled 'GOAL', that is Game Oriented Activities for Learning, and it is available in the UK from LDA, Wisbech, Cambs. PE13 2AX.) Level 1, which is devised for nursery and first year primary children, older ESN children and the mentally subnormal, consists of 337 lesson plans related to the psycholinguistic abilities identified and assessed by the ITPA. Lesson plans are graded and in addition a great deal of actual material such as puppets, jig-saw puzzles, cut out patterns and so forth, is included. Level 2 is similar, although it is designed for children over the age of 6 years and gives more emphasis to teaching related literacy skills. There is no doubt that this equipment is excellent for therapists and teachers and provides masses of actual material to help plan and implement therapy. However, it must be noted that the cost of this programme is considerable and many therapists and teachers may have to make do with a source book to help them plan remediation.

If this is the case, a highly recommended text has been produced by

Bush and Giles (1977). Although similar in format to the chapters in Kirk and Kirk (1971), far more detailed activities are suggested for each area. For example, the chapter on auditory association describes over fifty activities which can be used to remediate poor performance. These activities are graded as in Karnes' programme and provide an incomparable source of ideas for therapists and teachers to adapt to their own needs and particular situations.

It is important to note two main points about therapeutic programmes based on the ITPA. First, although specific cognitive abilities are isolated in order to undertake remediation, this does not mean that the subtests are not inter-related. Indeed, Kirk and Kirk (1971, p. 134) stress that 'the most effective remediation attempts to integrate the disability with other abilities'. This implies that children's cognitive strengths are able to compensate for their weaknesses and that therapy should be planned accordingly.

Secondly, because the model of the ITPA is based upon psycholinguistic abilities, this can lead to therapists over-emphasising remediation in these areas without relating them directly to language. It is likely that this kind of approach could undermine the potential value of the ITPA as a therapeutic tool. In contrast, Cooper *et al.* (1979) place considerable emphasis in their programme on the importance of linking language to cognitive behaviour.

The mass of published material based on the ITPA makes it a very attractive test from which to plan remediation. However, it is important for therapists or teachers to monitor carefully their performance and to change and adapt the material to the perceived needs of any particular child. As Kirk and Kirk (1971, p. 117) note 'diagnosis should be an ongoing process'. This also implies that therapy can never be static, a point which must be considered in evaluating the efficacy of remediation based on the ITPA.

Related Research

The ITPA has stimulated a great deal of research over the last decade, and is a good example of one attempt at psycholinguistic training. The effectiveness of this kind of approach has caused considerable debate and controversy in the literature and has led to quite extreme viewpoints. In many ways this is predictable, especially as the ITPA sets out to be a diagnostic test and to suggest approaches to remediation, unlike the Reynell which tends to be more descriptive.

Bloom and Lahey (1978, Chapter XIX) question whether deficient cognitive abilities cause language disorders or whether they result from language difficulties in the first place. They conclude that specific cognitive abilities may not be distinct from one another and that they do not appear to be prerequisites for language learning as there is no evidence that remediation in these areas improves general language functioning.

This conclusion was derived primarily from a review by Hammill and Larsen (1974) which raised a number of important issues and has also stimulated further debate. In this paper they reviewed the results of 38 studies from 1962 to 1974 which attempted to train children in psycholinguistic skills and used the ITPA as the criterion for improvement. Only studies in which there were comparisons between children receiving psycholinguistic training and those receiving no formal instruction or enrolled in 'traditional' programmes were included. From an extremely detailed analysis of these studies they argued that the idea that concepts as measured by the ITPA can be trained remains non-validated. They were unable to suggest whether this was because psycholinguistic abilities are difficult to teach and the training programmes inadequate, or whether it may have been that the ITPA is not sensitive enough to show any changes. The main implication drawn was that the efficacy of psycholinguistic training had not been conclusively demonstrated.

However, Lund, Foster and McCall-Perez (1978) re-evaluated the studies reviewed and the conclusions drawn by Hammill and Larsen (1974). They re-examined 24 studies which were divided into three; those showing positive results, those showing negative results and other studies. Positive results were those where there were gains on six or more of the subtests and on the overall total. This resulted in a total of 6 studies all showing positive results. There were 10 studies which Hammill and Larsen recorded as showing negative results, but Lund *et al.* argued that a re-examination of these demonstrates that 8 either showed equivocal or positive results. In examining the remaining studies, they suggested that 3 of them demonstrated positive gains on specifically selected subtests and that no firm conclusions could be drawn from the rest. They conclude that their examination of the original data reviewed by Hammill and Larsen, leads to a different conclusion, namely, that psycholinguistic training is feasible in some situations and not in others.

As would be expected Hammill and Larsen (1978) replied to Lund *et al.* reaffirming their original position. It becomes clear from this reply that the dispute is in part centred on methodological interpretations of what actually constitutes significant improvement. Hammill and Larsen place particular emphasis on the concept of statistical significance rather than on predetermined criteria for improvement. For example, whereas Lund *et al.* argue that improvement on one out of four subtests is a positive recommendation for psycholinguistic training, Hammill and Larsen suggest that this is not the case at all. Similar disputes arise concerning whether experimental groups should be compared to control groups or whether pre- and post-test measures of the experimental group are sufficient. Hammill and Larsen summarise by concluding that without further experimental validation they will remain doubtful about the viability of psycholinguistic training programmes.

Although psycholinguistic training is not necessarily based on the ITPA, and the two cannot be equated, the debate outlined above has important implications for evaluating the therapeutic approaches suggested by Kirk and Kirk (1971). It is almost impossible to come to any definite conclusion about the efficacy of psycholinguistic training. However, it seems likely that it is the particular circumstances and situational variables affecting any programme, which determine not only the actual effectiveness of remediation, but how different researchers, therapists and teachers come to judge the value of any given approach.

A good illustration of this is a British study conducted by Evesham (1977) and not mentioned in the above debate. In this study, children within 'normal limits of intelligence' needing special education and speech therapy because of specific language disabilities were used. These children were placed in a special class in a normal infants school and received one hour of therapy a day based on the ITPA. The rest of the time was spent as normal. These children were matched with a control group from another infants school, who were taught by 'traditional' teaching methods and given individual speech therapy. On the basis of pre- and post-treatment tests given at the beginning and end of the school year, Evesham found that the experimental group had made the most improvement in language ability. For example, statistically significant improvement for pre- to post-test scores was found for the experimental group on both the Comprehension and Expressive Scales of the Reynell. No statistically significant improvement was found for the control group. Evesham concluded that teaching language skills on the basis of the ITPA model is suitable for use with children in a Language Unit.

The results of this study are particularly interesting in the light of the above debate. It would be expected that Hammill and Larsen would conclude that this study could not be classed as successful, because no comparisons were made between the control and experimental groups. On the other hand, Lund *et al.* would count this study as successful as the experimental group demonstrated improvement on pre- to post-test measures.

A more reasonable viewpoint is that given the situation in which Evesham was working and the particular circumstances affecting the programme, it can be concluded that remediation was 'successful'. It clearly seemed to work for this set of children taught by a certain combination of teachers and speech therapists in this type of Language Unit. On the other hand, as pointed out by Evesham herself, the results are difficult to generalise to other samples of children who will be affected by a completely different set of variables, ranging from the personalities of the researchers to the nature of the school buildings.

There is clearly no black or white answer to the overall question of the effectiveness of psycholinguistic training, including programmes based on the ITPA, only various shades of grey depending upon the circumstances affecting any particular study. This is linked to the statement by Kirk and Kirk (1971) that diagnosis is an ongoing process and the consequent deduction that therapy cannot be static. The assumption which has to be made in research studies is that therapy is static and hence can be evaluated objectively. In reality this cannot be the case and if it were it would hinder rather than enhance therapy.

In a recent discussion of the uses and abuses of the ITPA, Kirk and Kirk (1978) conclude that tests cannot substitute for good observations and clinical judgements. In examining the efficacy of training based on the ITPA it may be that not only are therapeutic techniques being evaluated, but therapists and teachers as well. This important human 'variable' confounds all the reported research on the ITPA and makes it difficult, even pointless, to try to come to any definite generalisable conclusion.

Appraisal

The usefulness of the ITPA is extremely difficult to appraise. Whereas there has been little research on the Reynell and more is obviously needed, there has been a mass of data collected on the ITPA. However, as has already been pointed out, there is considerable disagreement on the value of psycholinguistic training and on the use of tests such as the ITPA as diagnostic tools to guide remediation. In a brief review Mittler (1976) suggests that the ITPA has in fact not fully lived up to expectations.

Certainly the theoretical model on which the ITPA is based appears to be out of date in the light of recent work on psycholinguistics. None of the research undertaken during the seventies appears to have been incorporated into the model or reflected in the test (see Bloom and Lahey, 1978 for a review). Similarly, the test suffers in comparison with, for example, the LARSP (Crystal *et al.*, 1976) by not including any assessment of children's linguistic abilities, to the extent that syntax is ignored completely. The auditory reception subtest is particularly weak, relying as it does on 'yes' or 'no' responses which is only a limited measure of auditory understanding.

However, the ITPA provides a wealth of potentially diagnostic information to guide remediation. As a tool for generating ideas and hypotheses about possible causes of language disorders, the ITPA is without equal. Its strength lies in that it is designed not to isolate language from general cognitive functioning, but in such a way as to enable therapists and teachers to gain broader perspectives on the factors affecting children's language disorders.

Unlike intelligence tests, the ITPA is diagnostic and hence attempts to provide causal explanations to guide remediation. In doing this it is more likely than not to be shown at some time to be wrong. But as knowledge increases, any model of language development which is being used, will eventually be shown to be wrong. This after all, is the way that science progresses. The advantage of the ITPA, is that it stimulates ideas and suggests therapeutic strategies which can be tried out and evaluated, and it is because of this that it is easier to question its usefulness than it is many other therapeutic approaches.

In conclusion, it is felt that the ITPA still has an important role to play in assessing language and in indicating remediation. Yet, the limitations of the test are recognised and it may be time for the ITPA to undergo further revision to reflect an ever increasing knowledge of psycholinguistics. Osgood's original model has probably outlived its usefulness and now needs modification in the light of recent findings in psychology and linguistics.

Aston Index

Theoretical Background

The Aston Index is a battery of tests put together by Newton and Thomson which is designed to identify children having difficulties with written language, especially those who might be suspected of being dyslexic. It is available in the UK from LDA, Wisbech, Cambs.

PE13 2AX.) Unlike the ITPA or the Reynell, the Index is not based on a particular psycholinguistic model of language development. Instead, it attempts to identify and assess the kind of classroom based skills which are necessary for the acquisition of reading, spelling and writing in order to provide a meaningful profile for the purpose of remediation. Although it is not a psycholinguistic test in the strict sense of the word, it does provide relevant information about a child's overall abilities relating to language performance.

Although specifically designed to identify dyslexic-type difficulties, the Aston Index is marketed as a classroom based test for the screening of 'language difficulties' in children aged from 5 to 14 years. In fact it is claimed that it can identify slow learners, the educationally subnormal and language disordered children. Consequently, the test is widely available to teachers, speech therapists and others with an interest in identifying children with learning difficulties.

Description and Administration

The Index is designed to assess both general and specific abilities. It can be administered at one of two levels. Level 1 is for children between the ages of 5 and 7 years. It is designed to examine those pre-reading skills which would seem to underlie later school achievement. Hence, the test items do not require the ability to read or write. The following subtests are included: Picture Recognition; a Vocabulary Scale; the Goodenough Draw-a-Man Scale; Copying Geometric Designs; a test of Laterality; Copying Name; Visual Sequential Memory (pictorial); Auditory Sequential Memory; Sound Blending; Visual Sequential Memory (symbolic); and Sound Discrimination. Most of these are taken from standardised tests of intelligence.

Level 2 is designed for children over the age of 7 years having general problems relating to reading, writing and language. It is comprised of the following subtests: the Stanford-Binet Vocabulary Scale; an Aston Vocabulary Scale; the Goodenough Draw-a-Man Scale; Copying Geometric Designs; the Schonell Graded Word Reading Test; the Schonell Graded Spelling Test; a test of Laterality; a test of Free Writing; Visual Sequential Memory (pictorial); Auditory Sequential Memory; Sound Blending; Visual Sequential Memory (symbolic); Sound Discrimination; a test of Grapheme/Phoneme Correspondence and a Graphomotor Test.

From this information, profiles of children's learning patterns can be drawn up and specific subtest results examined. If on the Draw-a-Man or Vocabulary Tests, a child scores a year or more below chronological age, further assessment of intelligence may be needed. It is suggested that children having difficulty with picture recognition, yet who do well on other mental age measures such as copying designs, may have expressive language difficulties. The reading and spelling tests help to identify particular patterns of errors, such as disordered word patterns (destart/desert) or bizarre spelling. From the memory tests, information about perceptual processing and in particular sequencing can be gained. Similarly, poor performance on the sound blending test reflects poor auditory sequencing. If a child receives poor scores on sound discrimination it is suggested that there is a need for audiometric assessment, although it should be noted that every child with speech and language problems should automatically have an audiometric examination. The rest of the tests assess motor ability and indicate whether the child may have laterality problems. Overall, the Aston enables a good picture to be built up of school based abilities related to the general development of language skills.

Standardised data is available for a sample of 683 school children in the West Midlands area (Newton, Thomson and Richards, 1979). Means, standard deviations and standard errors on most of the tests are given at six monthly intervals for children aged between 5½ and 10½ years. Correlations between the various test scores and some indication of the re-test reliability is also included. In using the Index, special care needs to be given to interpreting the test scores of children aged eleven years or older as there is limited standardised information available. Unlike the ITPA and to a lesser extent the Reynell, the Aston is still at a very early stage of development.

Therapeutic Implications and Related Research

Although the Aston Index has initiated a considerable amount of research, this has been directed almost entirely at the phenomenon of 'dyslexia' (Newton *et al.*, 1979). At the time of writing there are no norms or sample profiles readily available to enable children with language disorders to be identified. It is uncertain then, to what extent the Aston can diagnose and indicate remediation for children with language problems. The claim that it can distinguish particular problems and enable appropriate teaching programmes to be planned has yet to be demonstrated.

However, the Aston does give the same kind of guidelines for remediation as the ITPA, and it is not unreasonable to suggest that for children with learning disabilities, therapy might proceed along the lines suggested, for example, by Bush and Giles (1977). In a review of dyslexia therapy, Sampson (1976) notes the relevance of remediation derived from the ITPA. The emphasis in both tests given to sequencing and auditory processes reflects the importance of these skills for planning remediation programmes for children with language disorders. At this stage more research is needed to evaluate fully the usefulness of the Aston Index for children presenting with language difficulties.

Appraisal

In terms of availability, the potential use of the Aston is far greater than that of either the Reynell or the ITPA. As a screening test it is probably the best one available, both in terms of cost and ease of administration. It covers a wide variety of abilities which are clearly related to the skills of language. Although it only gives a general indication of these abilities, it points the way towards further and more detailed assessment. At the present time, the Aston Index is probably most useful to assess school based abilities and to serve as a complement to tests like the Reynell and the ITPA.

Conclusion

There has been little agreement about the exact role played by psycholinguistic abilities in the acquisition and use of language. The controversy arising from the claims that psycholinguistic deficiencies are either causal in the development of the skills of language, or are simply a reflection of poor language ability in the first place, is almost impossible to resolve. In fact it can be argued that the question itself is meaningless and that a simple one way relationship does not exist.

As noted in Chapter 1, a parallel argument has centred around the wider issue of the relationship between language and thought, and as pointed out earlier Bruner (1975) has put forward the idea that sometimes language determines thought and acts as a 'mould' and that at other times language can act as a 'cloak' and simply represent what is already known. It is further argued that to some extent individuals are able to choose how they use language depending upon the situation and their level of intellectual development.

This argument can profitably be extended to the current problem. It does not seem unreasonable to suggest that in some cases there are certain cognitive abilities underlying language performance. Comprehending conversation for example, clearly involves auditory short term memory and the general ability to sequence information. In other situations though, language itself is almost certainly the medium used to code information related to cognitive performance. For example, describing objects or recording certain information in short term memory, both involve the use of language to organise cognitive activity. Perhaps the difference between children with, and those without, learning disabilities, is that those without have learned to code information be it verbally or cognitively, and to some extent are in control of their behaviour. It may be that children with learning disabilities are incapable of selecting appropriate strategies to apply to different cognitive activities.

Finally, it must be emphasised that 'developmental psycholinguistic approaches' should be used in conjunction with other forms of assessment and remediation. In particular, for children having expressive problems including deviant language, the broad range of techniques discussed in Chapter 2 are invaluable. There is not just one approach which can be used exclusively in isolation from knowledge gathered in other fields of study, and therapists and teachers must exercise their professional judgement in selecting suitable forms of remediation from the wide range available.

4 CHILDHOOD BILINGUALISM

Chapter Outline

Some of the characteristics of bilingual speech highlighted have in the past been viewed as deficiencies but are now recognised as being acceptable within the bilingual environment. Difficulties of assessing the language development of bilinguals are described and suggestions made as to how to overcome these problems, sometimes relying on those very characteristics previously considered deviant in order to measure development. The need to consider both languages is stressed along with recognition of the child's possible bi-cultural situation. This emphasis on the two languages is continued where assessment is related to remediation.

Introduction

In the past, the term 'bilingual' has been criticised on the grounds of ambiguity, but here it is used specifically, and one hopes unambiguously, to refer to speakers of two 'distinct' languages. It does not encompass cases of diglossia, defined by Ferguson (1959) as 'two or more varieties of the same language'. Although it is not intended to enumerate and evaluate the various definitions of 'bilingual', it should be pointed out that it is a label which is wide-ranging in its applications. The definition forming the basis of this chapter will be 'the alternate use of two languages in the same individual'. While the vagueness of 'use' may run counter to the specificity professed above, it does avoid the problems arising from specification of quality as in Haugen's (1956) definition of bilingualism '. . . the ability to produce *complete* and *meaningful* utterances . . .' (italics added). The dangers are obvious when applied to developmental issues.

The logical distinction for structuring purposes would seem to be between simultaneous and sequential language acquisition, the former referring to the consistent exposure of a child to two languages before 3 years of age, the latter to exposure to a second language after 3 years. The discussion will be organised according to this distinction but will be restricted to the assessment of bilingual *children*.

Further restrictions are imposed for various reasons. First, although the determination of language dominance is seen as a first step in assessment, the methods devised for doing so are too numerous to be discussed here (see Jones, 1966). Secondly, the assessment and subsequent remediation of verbal comprehension problems in bilingual children is largely excluded, except in so far as comprehension cannot be ignored in any discussion about therapy, but in no way does this exclusion reflect the customary approach to communication problems. Many of the studies to date have taken into account the bilingual's *output*, and as the aim of this chapter is to apply existing knowledge to the areas of assessment and remediation, it would be uneconomical to speculate at length on possible avenues of research related to verbal comprehension in bilingual children.

The approach then is based on selectivity, and attempts to pick out useful principles and techniques from the general field of research into bilingualism rather than to advocate any particular approach.

Simultaneous Acquisition

Even in monolingual communities, where there are relatively clear norms of development, language assessment is not a simple procedure. In bilingual areas, variations in type and degree of exposure to target languages further complicate the issue, making it difficult to obtain meaningful norms in the traditional sense. Apart from the problems of collating norms for each of the bilingual's languages (Munro, 1979) it may be argued that young, incipient bilinguals do not in fact possess separate sets of norms, their languages developing in a unified rather than an independent manner. In addition, there is variability in the timing of divergence of the two languages, after which point there is likely to be continued intrusion between them.

What emerges therefore is a need to assess firstly the child's abilities in language A as compared with bilingual peers; secondly, the child's abilities in language B, again with reference to the linguistic environment; and thirdly, the child's total communicative competence, using languages A and B together (see Abudarham, 1980, on vocabulary testing). Only in this way can it be ensured that treatment is actually indicated and, if so, pinpoint those problems affecting both languages in addition to those which are language-specific.

One of the first steps in assessment is to eliminate those characteristics which are not problems in a 'clinical' sense. When any two languages develop together in the one individual it is customary for interference to take place. Though controversy continues as to its value in explaining learner error in sequential acquisition, it is evident that patterns occur in simultaneous language learning which can only be attributed to the presence of a two-language system. However, reports on degrees of interference in these children differ widely, varying not only between authors but also according to the level of language (phonological, syntactic or semantic) referred to. In this chapter interference is considered to be the simultaneous application of the patterns of two languages to the same item, e.g. the construction 'littleaf' (smallest) containing the English stem 'little' and Welsh superlative affix '-af'. It does not include the phenomenon of lexical borrowing where a word from language A is used with little or no modification in language B and may even become an accepted item in the latter's lexicon; again exemplifying from Welsh-English bilingualism –

> 'Mae'r *garage* yn fach'
> Is the garage in small (The garage is small)

What is difficult, especially for the monlingual assessor, is recognising that, on the whole, interference is the rule rather than the exception in early bilingual development and then deciding which utterances are the result of that interference. That is not to say that any amount of interference is acceptable; in the absence of norms for bilingual development one can only speculate about the quality and quantity permissible at each developmental stage. However, if one recognises that it is a characteristic of the norm, then interference, like other aspects of language behaviour, becomes a potential means of measuring delayed development. When immaturities in interference patterns can be recognised it is possible to start to pinpoint deviations, that is, utterances which can be attributed to confusion between two languages but are not confusions which fit into a normal developmental sequence for bilinguals.

Of course, interference is not the only characteristic of simultaneous bilingualism which can be used to measure delay. Another potential area is development of the child's *awareness* of distinguishable modes of spoken language. Unfortunately, the age at which a bilingual child is said to become conscious of the existence of two different languages varies dramatically. This is an issue dealt with more thoroughly by McLaughlin (1978) where it is explained that the variations arise from the use of different criteria for 'awareness'. Workable and consistent measures would be useful, particularly as it could be argued that this differentiation of languages is related to interference – that it is difficulty with the former that leads to the latter. In therapeutic terms, this is a significant link for it suggests a means of dealing with 'excessive' interference by developing the child's consciousness of the two languages, rather than resorting to elimination of one of them in order to solve the problem. At the early stage of naming, for instance, a concept introduced via a language A label could be reinforced by its equivalent label from language B, added prominence being given to one or other label if it is more useful or usual in that particular language. Introduction of labels without equivalents in the other language would be determined by the needs of the child. The principle underlying this approach is based on the findings of the more recent studies on bilingual development and education (for example, Davies, 1979) which stress the advantages for children of a two-language system. They claim that the bilingual environment increases the child's perception of the world and renders him better able to analyse language as an abstract system. There is a need to investigate more fully the positive aspects of bilingualism in linguistically normal children and their possible applications to therapy with the language impaired.

There is a need also to take into account peculiarities of bilingual speech, other than interference, which some assessors erroneously think signify a need for intervention. One illustration is that of code alternation which involves the use of successive stretches of two languages (see Table 4.1) often giving the impression that the speaker lacks control of the structural systems of the two languages and is mixing them indiscriminately. In fact, not only is this alternation common in bilingual speech, but according to Dulay, Hernández-Chávez and Burt (1978)* it 'obeys rather strict structural rules in addition to the grammatical rules of each of the component languages' (p. 295). These rules ensure that code alternation occurs at specific, definable syntactic junctures, each unilingual section retaining an internal consistency characteristic of monlingual grammar and phonology. (See also Lindholm and Padilla, 1978; Pfaff, 1979.) Although Dulay *et al.* give only tentative guidelines regarding the determinants of natural code alternation, they are useful in assessment for they begin to provide a framework whereby we can evaluate the child's ability to obey what Dulay and his co-authors refer to as 'a set of intersystemic wellformedness conditions' (p. 296). Table 4.1 indicates some of the junctures cited by them as being permissible alternation points.

*These authors include examples of utterances which relate to the present description of lexical borrowing. Their interpretation of the term 'code alternation' is therefore less specific.

Table 4.1: Examples of Acceptable Code Alternation

Juncture	Illustration	Source of Illustration
1. At relative clause boundary	'You know my brother *a aeth i'r Brifysgol*'. ('You know my brother who went to the University')	English-Welsh Adult Speech. Own data
2. Before adverbial clause	'The type of work he did, *cuando trabajaba*, he . . .' ('The type of work he did, when he worked, he . . .')	English-Spanish Adult Speech (Gumperz and Hernández-Chávez, 1971)
3. At beginning of verb phrase	'And my uncle Sam *es el mas agabachado*' ('And my uncle Sam is the most Americanised')	English-Spanish Adult Speech (Dulay *et al.*, 1978)

Needless to say one cannot apply these adult standards to bilingual children of all ages. The ability to apply rules of alternation, while maintaining the internal consistency previously referred to, is precluded by the conscious separation of the codes into discrete languages. Thus, we return to the necessity for establishing ages at which different types of bilinguals ('balanced' as well as one-language dominant) achieve code differentiation.

The evaluation of bilingual speech, whether it be of the limited language differentiation causing interference or the higher degree of differentiation involved in code alternation, should not be done from a monolingual standpoint. Admittedly, in monolingual situations, such phenomena may be said to limit communication, but it is maintained that the output can be fairly assessed only if one considers the bilingual input to which the child is subjected. This is a difficult task rendered even harder by the paucity of standardised tests for bilingual children and, therefore, an assessor often has to rely on samples of free speech as a basis for assessment. For instance, omitting cases of code alternation, a syntactic analysis may be carried out as suggested in Figure 4.1. Even when the languages of a bilingual community are consistently A and B, analysis such as the above, which requires a working knowledge of both languages, is demanding in terms of time and skill. When assessing in an area where the children are reared to speak languages A + B, or A + C, or A + D . . ., it is clear that an individual is unlikely to possess the expertise required to analyse not only the separate languages but also the various ways in which they interact. One solution to the problem is the creation of a community-based assessment team, the members of which, between them, can provide detailed information about the structure and development of the languages occurring simultaneously in that area.

Figure 4.1: Flowchart to Establish Sentence Structure Acceptability in Bilingual Children (Excluding Code Alternation)

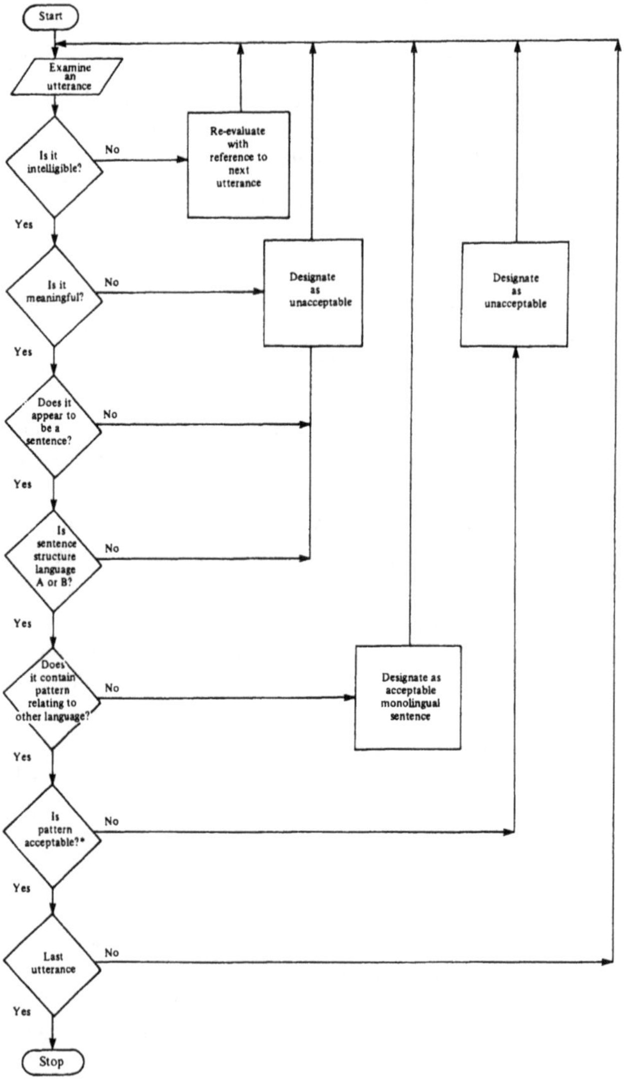

*With reference to language dominance/exposure and chronological age

Regardless of the number of assessors involved, the main aims of assessment remain the same – to demonstrate the need for remediation and provide guidelines for the planning of that remediation. Where assessment, resulting from the 'pooling' of information on both languages, uncovers common core deficits, a unified approach to therapy is indicated. Such an approach is based on the assumption that certain operating principles underlie the process of language learning and lend a natural structure to an intervention programme for bilinguals. Cross-linguistic studies and the search for language universals have provided information about the common properties of languages (Lieb, 1975; Greenberg, 1978; Sampson, 1978), but despite the fact that some of the generalisations arising from these studies suggest bases for remediation, very few have actually been developed with reference to language pathology.

Leaving aside the sometimes complex arguments concerning the relationship between cognitive and linguistic universals (see for example, McNeill, 1970 and Slobin, 1973), it is possible to mention here a *few* of the characteristics claimed to be virtually universal in human (child) language. They provide an insight into children's strategies for organising language(s) which could prove to be useful 'anchors' in therapy for children trying to cope with several communication systems. For instance, at the phonological level, it has been suggested that all children during the second year of life show a preference for consonant-vowel (CV) and occasional vowel-consonant (VC) sequences. Stops are generally acquired before fricatives, and there is a gradual development of phonemic perception beginning with vowel distinctions (see Ingram, 1976). At the syntactic level, at the earliest stage of development, children of different language backgrounds seem to work on the expression of subject-verb-object (SVO) relationships, in the combination SV, VO and, less commonly, SO. Other patterns, ordered according to the languages spoken, are noun-locative, adjective-noun and demonstrative pronoun-noun (see Bowerman, 1973).

In the search for such common properties one should not lose sight of the individuality of each language. As the child's linguistic forms are a reflection of his perception of relationships and an expression of underlying concepts, it is perhaps not surprising that there are similarities across languages. Nevertheless, the linguistic device employed to mark a particular notion may be more complex in one language than the other, thus affecting the order of its acquisition. Mikěs (1967) cites the example of Serbo-Croatian-Hungarian bilingual children who demonstrated locative relationships in Hungarian earlier than in

Serbo-Croatian. In the former language, the locative marker is expressed by noun inflection whereas in the latter a preposition is needed in addition to the noun inflection.

Thus, during the planning of remediation one has to take into account not only the likenesses between languages but also those specific differences which will affect the order in which some forms are introduced to the child.

Sequential Acquisition

If a child is learning English as a second language (i.e. after three years of age, having been exposed only to his native language) it is hardly surprising that the child's proficiency in English does not equal that of peers whose English is their first and perhaps only language. The sequential learner is particularly likely to give a poor impression of verbal ability if assessed only in English and at a time when the child has had little experience of that medium. In such a situation it can be difficult for the assessor to distinguish between inadequacies in English which are due purely to the 'foreign language' context and those resulting from a true pathology. The former context is likely to affect only (or mostly) the 'new' language whereas the effects of the latter will be witnessed in both languages. This fact highlights the need to assess the child in the two languages as it is only in this way that decisions can safely be made regarding the most suitable therapeutic programme to implement, whether it should be biased towards English as a second language or directed on a certain pathological problem.

Edwards (1979) points out that immigrant and ethnic group youngsters of limited English speaking ability enter school with a 'well functioning language system which is, simply, not that of the school' (p. 136). English-medium tests are unlikely to reveal this level of functioning in the native system thereby forfeiting valuable information about the child's total communicative ability. An Asian child, for instance, may not be using prepositions in English but be seen to use the equivalent post-positions in the native tongue. The child has the concept of spatial relations and a means of expressing them, thus presenting a different problem from the child with poor perceptual skills which affect any and all languages attempted. The relevance of this distinction for remediation is obvious.

In the past researchers have attempted to relate the errors of second language (L2) learners to the structure of their native language (L1).

Nowadays, however, the emphasis lies more on the similarities between the difficulties of L2 learners and the developmental errors of monolingual children (see following). Although this latter viewpoint reduces the importance of interference as a source of error, at least in sequential learning, it is not denied that relationships exist between the two languages. As exposure to L2* increases, these relationships may become more obvious. As English gains dominance the child may well 'borrow' from it, conversely, because dominance entails increasing demands on linguistic ability, the child may need to supplement English expressions with items from his L1. This has implications for assessment because:

(i) there is a need to assess not only his L1 and L2 but also the manner in which they combine. By this means one can evaluate the child's use of interlinguistic rules which, it is suggested, are indicative of creative abilities and thus language learning potential;
(ii) one needs to determine whether these patterns of interaction are characteristic of that child's bilingual community.

In analysing languages which combine in some way with one another, there is a tendency to rely on monolingual tests, but these are unlikely to produce realistic and useful profiles, particularly where the degree of inter-relating results in the child speaking what Miller (1978) refers to as 'an interlanguage'. Miller advocates a study of the child's sociolinguistic background in order to decide on the language most appropriate for the comprehension and/or expression of the content of a particular test. The test is then administered in that language, but if the subject fails to respond, the item is repeated in the other language, thereby gaining some impression of 'collective competence'. Of course, it must be ensured that the response given to the repeated item is indeed equivalent to that expected for the original item. This can be difficult as structural or semantic equivalence between languages need not be synonymous with equivalent *order* of acquisition of those structures or meanings. For instance, a word in one language may develop later than its semantic equivalent in the other language, depending on the relative importance of that word in the culture of each linguistic group.

Whether one is assessing the two languages separately or together, this lack of correspondence has a detrimental effect on the suitability of items which are merely translations from techniques devised in other

*In this chapter L2 refers to English, unless otherwise specified.

languages. Direct translation also fails to take account of the fact that some of the concepts common in Language A may be unfamiliar to the culture of Language B.

Even if provided with details of the order and nature of acquisition of languages other than English, the assessor is faced with the problem of pronouncing test items in a language foreign to him. Also, decisions have to be made on the acceptability of responses which are neither completely right nor wrong. Many assessors have resorted to using interpreters but it is not easy to obtain objective individuals who also have some knowledge of language development. One solution to the pronunciation aspect is the use of foreign language tests, tape-recorded by native speakers of those languages. Unfortunately, the adequate evaluation of the child's responses in his L1 remains an unsolved problem in many cases.

Although evaluation of the child's L2 is usually less problematic, it is not easy to decide on the significance of the patterns appearing in English: are they typical of delayed development; is the delay related to the degree of exposure to English; if atypical, are the patterns in any way connected to the structure of the L1? Assessment in this area can be assisted by considering the evidence supporting the hypothesis that L2 progresses through stages similar to monolingual L1 development (for example, Ervin-Tripp, 1974 and Milon, 1974). Such evidence suggests that the learning of English as an L2 shows striking parallels with native English acquisition. This enables the assessor to apply information about L1 learning to L2 situations and therefore to gauge whether the child is applying suitable language processing strategies, and to decide if these processes are developing in the expected order. These similarities between English L1 development and L2 learning of English are maintained across groups of differing native languages, as exemplified in Tables 4.2 and 4.3. This means that an assessment modelled on the acquisition sequence of certain functions in L2 English can be used on children of various L1 backgrounds.

There are implications for management too. Hatfield (1979) studied the English learning of 31 Punjabi and Chinese speaking children in Glasgow and found a high correlation between both groups for the acquisition order of eight English morphemes. She then related her findings to existing methods of teaching English as a second language and discovered a discrepancy between what was taught and what was produced in spontaneous speech. The practice of withdrawing bilingual children for structured drilling was felt to be counter-productive because learning a second language is a creative process whereby the learner works out hypotheses about that system, much as a child learns his first language. Thus, Hatfield advocates:

(i) a 'total' language environment;
(ii) that the child's cultural background be emphasised rather than ignored;
(iii) that teaching methods approximate to the way small children develop in natural settings.

Although these points relate to teaching those children who presumably have no difficulties with their L1, they are relevant to other professions such as Speech Therapy as they focus on acquisition and education in normal (bilingual) groups, so often the starting point for developing techniques for remediation.

Table 4.2: Wh – Questions
Characteristic noted in L2: early inability to invert auxiliary verb and subject.

L.1	L.2	Source
Norwegian	English	Ravem (1974)
French	English	Ervin-Tripp (1974)

Table 4.3: Negation
Stages noted in L2:
(i) negative appears outside sentence nucleus
(ii) negative appears between noun phrase and verb phrase
(iii) adult pattern

L.1	L.2	Source
Spanish	English	Hernández-Chávez (1972)
Norwegian	English	Ravem (1974)
Japanese	English	Milon (1974)

Such studies do not claim that second language learning is simply a recapitulation of early language acquisition. Different cognitive skills are involved. Furthermore, the uniformity in learning patterns is not absolute, variations arise due to different timing of exposure to the L2. Also, one must consider those variations due to interference and the problems they present for assessment, some of which have already been discussed. As in simultaneous bilingualism, a certain amount of interference is natural but dependence on L1 structures may become more prevalent in children who have basic problems of language differentiation and formulation. Bearing in mind that L2 learners tend to show patterns typical of younger monolingual children, it can be hard to determine whether a response is an immature form or an example of interference. For instance, a Welsh speaking child of five years, learning English, might respond to the question 'What is she doing?' with the word, 'run'. Failure to include the present participle '-ing' in this elided sentence could be a delay in mastering the correct morpheme in English. Alternatively, it could be due to a generalisation from the Welsh where the correct form 'rhedeg' is formed by the verb-noun with no suffix. A decision can only be made by relating to the corpus of data as a whole, that is, by searching for utterances which would not usually be found in monolingual children, thus excluding immaturity, or looking for those utterances which can not be attributed to interference and are therefore more clearly immature forms.

This type of analysis is in accord with other approaches to assessment proposed in this chapter for it moves away from the tendency to evaluate factors in isolation. In advocating such a 'total' approach, one should not forget the child's cultural background. Khan (1980) writing about linguistic minorities, suggests that if we are to find the most effective ways of realising their educational potential, 'we must start from the actual situation in which the children find themselves in society' (p. 76). We are not so much concerned here with the culture-specific language forms previously discussed but rather with issues such as appraisal of parental attitude to language, assessing the environmental demands upon the child's languages, and use of culture-free material for testing.

As assessment forms the basis to remediation, acquisition of such knowledge is important. Some of the cultural differences can actually hinder remediation. For instance, there are variations in attitudes towards dealing with developmental problems, where some ethnic groups are unworried by poor language development in the early years, or where there may be different expectations for male and female children. Only by being fully aware of these differences can one ensure that management of the case is realistically geared to the situation. The type of advice given to parents will obviously depend on the presenting problem. If the child is displaying difficulties in both languages and is mixing them indiscriminately, the therapist may need to explain the necessity for 'strict, predictable code differentiation' (Miller, 1978, p. 20). One structures the child's environment so that he is required to relate one language to one speaker, situation or topic. This is not a new concept. Ronjat (1913) and Smith (1935) both felt that it was best for children to receive two languages from different sources, consistently.

Advice may extend to counselling parents regarding their own learning of English. As the children bring English into the home from school, parents sometimes attempt to pick it up from their offspring. The poor L2 model which often results can do little to help a child already struggling, and in addition, his exposure to L1 is reduced.

Finally, it should be mentioned that reading, as a type of language assessment, must be adopted with caution. Edwards (1976) found that West Indian and English 11- and 12-year olds of similar social class and school ability were apparently equal in reading ability. However, the West Indians' comprehension of what was read was significantly less. This caution may be generalised to remediation contexts where reading is used as an opportunity for developing language in older L2 learners. Advances in actual reading ability need not signify an improved grasp of the underlying concepts.

Conclusion

In this chapter the argument has been put forward against the predisposition to assess bilingual children from a monolingual standpoint. For many years researchers (e.g. Macnamara, 1966 and Lloyd, 1977) concentrated on proving the disadvantages of bilingualism for verbal and non-verbal development, but the studies were frequently poorly designed, neglected to consider the part played by those social factors characteristic of bilingual groups and tended to look in detail at only one of the child's languages. Nevertheless, the techniques adopted influenced the way in which bilingual children were to be assessed, there being a preference for using unilingual tests. More recently however, research has highlighted the positive aspects, such as the greater cognitive flexibility of a two-language system. It is suggested here that in assessment such advantages should be capitalised upon rather than ignored. This can only be done if both languages and their combined use are considered.

It is not surprising that those studies which affected assessment methods have also had an effect on remediation. Apart from the fact that therapists and teachers have had to ignore languages unfamiliar to them, misconceptions about the ill-effects of a bilingual upbringing have led to situations where even those personnel who are themselves bilingual have chosen to work via one medium only. Others have advised parents to deny their child access to two languages. Of late, due to the more enlightened views on bilingualism, professionals concerned with remediation have attempted to plan programmes which cater for the unique needs of bilingual children and have striven to give realistic advice to parents as has been illustrated.

The marriage of complex areas such as assessment, remediation and bilingualism has created a need for simplification. It is suggested that this might be achieved by investigating more fully language universals and cross-linguistic similarities which may be adopted as guidelines to both assessment and remediation.

Finally, it must be said that there are likely to be language impaired children who will be unable to develop two languages. Unfortunately, our present state of knowledge is such that we are not always able to predict which children:

(i) will be totally confused by a second language;
(ii) will acquire certain aspects of both languages but in a fragmented fashion;
(iii) will manage to develop two 'workable' languages;
(iv) will positively benefit from exposure to more than one language.

Much analysis remains to be done of the language problems of bilingual children so that their assessment and subsequent remediation have a more secure basis than at present. However, a positive start has been made by the very recognition of the advantages of bilingualism.

5 ASSESSING ADULT APHASIA FOR REMEDIATION

Chapter Outline

This chapter discusses some principles and problems of aphasia testing and the clinical relevance of five major assessments of adult aphasia. These tests are The Minnesota Test for Differential Diagnosis of Aphasia, The Boston Diagnostic Aphasia Examination, The Porch Index of Communicative Ability, The Functional Communication Profile and The Token Test and Reporter's Test. Each test has its strengths and weaknesses from the clinical standpoint and assesses from different theoretical stances, placing emphasis on description and measurement of different aspects of adult aphasia. Consequently, each test provides qualitatively different kinds of information which may be useful in forming a basis for making clinical decisions.

Introduction

A non-controversial definition of adult aphasia might be that it is a disorder of language that can manifest itself through any mode of language, e.g. speech, reading, writing, and can affect receptive as well as expressive language and is a result of cerebral damage to those areas of the human brain which are responsible for processing higher cortical functions which underlie language.

Our knowledge of the relationships between brain function and language is minimal, and there is no single universally accepted theory which explains adequately the breakdown of language which characterises aphasia. Furthermore, there is still not available an aphasia assessment battery which is primarily based upon linguistic principles (Lesser, 1978; Whitaker and Whitaker, 1979). This may be due in part to the failure of linguistics to provide an adequate explanation of aphasic language beyond a purely descriptive framework (Farmer and O'Connell, 1979). Some of the tests discussed in this chapter are based upon theoretical notions of aphasic breakdown (the Boston Test and the Minnesota Test for Differential Diagnosis of Aphasia), while others claim to assess from a standpoint of purely objective observation (the Porch Index of Communicative Abilities and the Functional Communication Profile).

Goodglass and Kaplan (1972) point out that the assessment of aphasia may be undertaken for any one of three general reasons: to detect and classify an aphasia type which may provide indications as to localisation of the underlying brain lesion; to determine a performance level on particular linguistic skills to provide a baseline against which to detect change over time; and to assess the deficits and retained abilities of the patient in order to provide a basis for therapy. It is the latter of these aims of assessment which is of most concern for rehabilitation, although both the other aims of assessment have relevance for the clinician.

The tests to be discussed below are all very different. The structure, scoring and emphasis on different aspects of aphasic behaviour in a test, may be chosen to evaluate and exemplify particular features of aphasia, and perhaps to support particular theoretical assumptions about aphasia. The aim they all have in common, however, is some kind of quantitative and/or qualitative estimation of aphasic behaviour. As Wallace (1964) has pointed out, the *quantification* of responses gives levels of attainment on particular tasks and allows for the measurement of change on subsequent re-test, whereas the *qualitative* or diagnostic features of a test purport to say something about *the way* a patient is failing and, to some extent, *why* the patient is failing. Qualitative assessment attempts to determine those aspects of a patient's total problem which are contributing to failure on a specific task. The qualitative aspects of a test should help to provide indications as to the fundamental processes underlying a patient's failures, and therefore suggest possible therapeutic strategies which the clinician might employ.

The concern of this chapter is to examine the clinical usefulness of the tests discussed. Consequently, the following tests were selected because they were considered to be the most widely used in aphasia rehabilitation and to provide the most relevant information for clinical purposes: The Minnesota Test for Differential Diagnosis of Aphasia (Minnesota); The Boston Diagnostic Aphasia Examination (Boston); The Porch Index of Communicative Abilities (PICA); The Functional Communication Profile (FCP); The Token (TT) and Reporter's Tests (RT).

An important point that must be made before discussion proceeds, is that assessment should not be seen as something that is done once and put aside until the time arrives for the next test. Sparks (1978) has emphasised that assessment should be an on-going process where the clinician is constantly updating his or her appraisal of the patient's abilities.

This chapter will discuss the general strengths and weaknesses of the tests mentioned above with special consideration given to clinical applicability. For excellent general discussion of principles and specific approaches to aphasia therapy see Eisenson (1973) and Jenkins, Jiménez-Pabón, Shaw and Sefer (1975).

The Minnesota Test for Differential Diagnosis of Aphasia (Minnesota)

Theoretical Background

The Minnesota is one of the most popular aphasia batteries available, having been developed by Schuell and her associates over a number of years. The following discussion will be based on the second edition of *Schuell's Aphasia in Adults* (Jenkins, Jiménez-Pabón, Shaw and Sefer, 1975) published after Schuell's death by her colleagues and the second edition of *Differential Diagnosis of Aphasia with the Minnesota Test* (Schuell, 1973; revised by Sefer).

The Minnesota takes as its basis for testing a system of classification which is claimed to be descriptive and predictive and derived from longitudinal observations of a large population of aphasic subjects. The view that there are mutually exclusive types of aphasia is rejected: symptoms change in individual patients and classifications based upon the most obvious presenting symptoms will therefore be less successful in description and prediction. Similarly, Schuell and her associates reject the notion of an expressive-receptive dichotomy, which serves as the basis for some models of aphasia. Aphasia is seen as a uni-dimensional disorder, which in its 'pure' form entails a reduction in available vocabulary and an impairment in auditory verbal retention span which is evident in all modalities without specific perceptual or apraxic involvement.

This *pure* aphasic element is basic to all seven of the diagnostic and prognostic categories of aphasic impairment which Schuell describes. The different categories are characterised by varying degrees of apraxic, perceptual and motor complications in addition to the fundamental reduction in available vocabulary and impaired auditory verbal retention span.

The seven patterns of aphasic impairment, which it is claimed are obtainable from Minnesota results, are presented here in order of increasing severity. Simple aphasia, which is the pure form, is characterised by the primary aphasic symptoms of reduced available vocabulary and impaired auditory verbal retention span, and has an excellent prognosis. Aphasia with visual involvement, which can be seen as simple aphasia plus a complicating impairment of discrimination, recognition and recall of visual symbols, also has an excellent prognosis, but reading and writing improve less quickly. The next category is mild aphasia with persisting dysfluency, where a mild, simple aphasia is combined with a verbal apraxia which causes disintegrated and unco-ordinated articulation, and is worse when conscious control is relaxed; here also the aphasic element has an excellent prognosis. Patients with aphasia with scattered findings have a moderate degree of aphasic impairment which may be complicated by dysarthria and visual involvement; recovery may be limited due to confounding physiological and psychological factors. In aphasia with sensorimotor involvement, a severe aphasia is observed accompanied by a verbal apraxia; a good functional recovery is often achieved. Aphasia with intermittent auditory imperception involves severe aphasia and severe auditory processing difficulties; a functional but limited recovery is usually made. The seventh category is the irreversible aphasic syndrome where the patient has a global communication problem manifested in all modalities. The prognosis is very poor, with linguistic abilities never reaching functional adequacy.

Description and Administration

The Minnesota package consists of test record booklets, a test manual, the monograph *Differential Diagnosis of Aphasia with the Minnesota Test* and two sets of stimulus cards in 'flip' form. The test itself consists of 47 subtests – 9 under an auditory disturbances section; 9 under a visual and reading disturbances section; 15 under speech and language disturbances; 10 under visuomotor disturbances and 4 under disturbances of numerical relationships and arithmetic processes. Subtests within each section are hierarchically arranged in increasing order of difficulty, so that, for instance, the subtests in the visuomotor disturbances section range from copying Greek letters to writing a paragraph.

The test is scored on a plus-minus basis and subtest scores are expressed in terms of number of errors. The battery is comprehensive in so far as linguistic performance at all levels in all modalities is covered, with the notable exception of gesture and pantomime. Although the scoring method is plus-minus, and there are limitations to this method of scoring, it is suggested that the tester makes additional notes on performance during testing. Any additional qualitative remarks are not included in the final score, however, and a great deal of potentially important information is consequently ignored. The subtest scores can be summarised in the booklet in list form, and a category rating scale is provided of 0-6 for understanding, speech, reading, writing and dysarthria, which may be completed by the examiner. In addition, there is a diagnostic rating scale to aid classification, which rates 12 language abilities from 0-4. These rating scales are often not completed, although they can provide a useful summary of the patient's abilities. Indeed, classification of aphasia is difficult with the Minnesota without reference to the diagnostic rating scale. Schuell (Jenkins *et al.*, 1975) states that the course of recovery in aphasia cannot be predicted before the patient becomes neurologically stable and she suggests that a period of three months post-onset should have elapsed before testing on the Minnesota, as categories are subject to fluctuation before this time lapse.

Therapeutic Implications

Jenkins *et al.* (1975) in the second edition of *Schuell's Aphasia in Adults* devote four chapters to therapy with aphasic patients, and this still constitutes one of the most theoretically well developed approaches to aphasia rehabilitation. Much of what is said expounds the attitudes and assumptions of the developers of the Minnesota and the principles of aphasia therapy are firmly rooted in the general philosophy of the authors. The book contains a great deal of useful information, good sense and common humanity. It gives general guidelines and describes techniques for specific forms of impairment revealed by the Minnesota.

From the clinical point of view, the predictive capability of the Minnesota is the main strength of the test, but this is weakened by the requirement that it should not be administered before three months post-onset if reliable prediction of recovery is required. Other tests do not make this stipulation and are not dependent upon neurological stability before making a prognosis (e.g. the PICA). In practice, many clinicians will want to assess before three months post-onset in order to determine prognosis, make clinical decisions and plan treatment. Gallaher (1979) tested 15 subjects three times over an eight day period with the Token Test less than three months post-onset and found high test-retest reliability. This indicates that stability may be established earlier than three months post-onset for most aphasic patients.

The test assesses ability in a wide range of linguistic skills in the major modalities at all levels of difficulty, and should highlight specific areas of deficit for treatment. However, it is weak in its analysis and presentation of test results.

Related Research

Like many aphasia batteries, the Minnesota has been criticised for its length and a number of shortened versions have been developed (Schuell, 1957; Schuell, 1966; Thompson and Enderby, 1979; Powell, Bailey and Clark, 1980). Schuell's (1966) re-evaluation of her own shortened version suggested to her that a short form cannot provide sufficient information upon which to make a diagnosis because it does not cover a large enough sample of language behaviour; test reliability being to some degree a function of test length. She suggests instead that an alternative strategy to reduce testing time is to select the highest test item that the tester considers the patient can pass without error in a particular modality. If the patient makes just one error on the subtest selected, the tester goes back to the next easiest item and starts again. This strategy has the advantage of cutting out the easiest items where the patient will presumably make no errors.

The short version developed by Thompson and Enderby (1979) analysed the full Minnesota results of 88 subjects. They conducted an item analysis to determine which subtests of the full test were redundant because they were either too easy or too difficult and therefore of minimal value in discriminating between patients. Having established which items of the full test were the most discriminative, they selected these new items for inclusion in the short version. High positive correlations of above 0.9 between these new items and the items from the full version were obtained, suggesting that this short form with only five items in each subtest and a revised scoring scale, produces similar test patterns to the full Minnesota. The scores can be transferred to a profile sheet (Figure 5.1) which includes Section Score Summary and percentile ranks established on the 88 subjects used in the trials.

This move towards shortening aphasia tests in general, and the Minnesota in particular, has recently resulted in a *very* short version of Schuell's test (Powell, Bailey and Clark, 1980). This screening test consists of one subtest taken from each of the first four sections of the full Minnesota. Subtest A4 (identifying items named serially), B8 (oral reading, words), C13 (naming pictures) and D6 (written spelling) were selected on the basis that they correlated more highly with the section they represented than with any other section and that they correlated with each other as little as possible. They were also the shortest subtests in the Minnesota, the most easily scored and required the minimum of special materials. With this very short screening version high positive correlations of greater than 0.9 were obtained between the short and full versions of the test. A result of rejecting more difficult subtests of

Figure 5.1: Assessment Summary Form of the Shortened Minnesota (Thompson and Enderby, 1979)

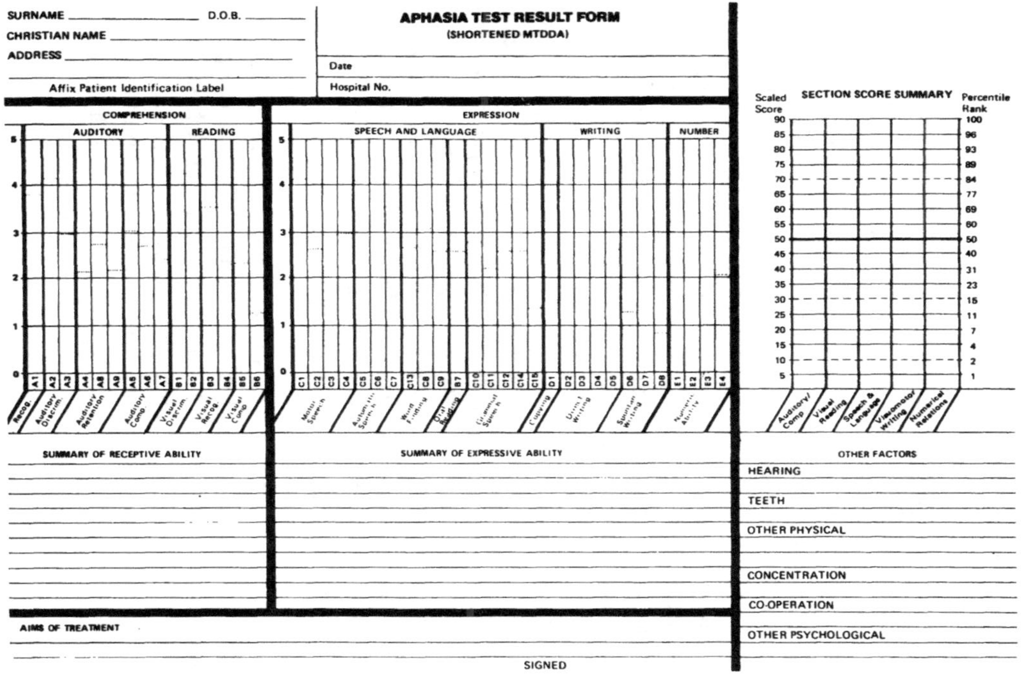

Source: Reproduced with special permission of Pam Enderby, Chief Speech Therapist, Frenchay Hospital, Bristol.

the Minnesota does mean that this very short test misclassified some milder aphasic patients amongst the 86 subjects tested (13 per cent of the sample were misclassified). Clearly this very short test (which takes less than 15 minutes to administer) makes no attempt to do more than *detect* aphasia, but this in itself may be useful as a screening procedure administered before time is invested on fuller assessment for planning therapy.

Support for the general theoretical basis of the Minnesota is suggested by a factor analysis of the test scores of 155 aphasic subjects carried out by Schuell, Jenkins and Carroll (1962). This study resulted in the identification of five factors, the first of which was interpreted to mean that there is a non-modality specific general language deficit in aphasia. Reading and writing deficits due to visual discrimination disturbances, impairment of the perception of spatial relationships, a dysarthric element and an apraxic element were also revealed by the analysis. The results and interpretation of this study does provide some support for the view that aphasia is a uni-dimensional general language deficit with added perceptual and motor complications.

Clark, Crockett and Klonoff (1979a), in their factor analysis of PICA scores, isolated a 'general or higher order language impairment factor' (p. 5) which they considered to be consistent with Schuell's view that there is a general hierarchy of language impairment common to all types of aphasia. However, Goodglass has pointed out (Goodglass and Geschwind, 1976; Goodglass and Kaplan, 1972; Goodglass, Quadfasel and Timberlake, 1964) that factor analysis of test scores of large groups of unselected severe aphasic patients is bound to result in the isolation of a general language factor.

Powell, Clark and Bailey (1979) subjected the Minnesota scores of 86 subjects to cluster analysis to determine if there was statistical validity for Schuell's subjective classification of seven categories of aphasia. The results revealed just four groups of aphasic subjects differing along a severity continuum – a severe, high moderate, low moderate and mild group. These results do not confirm the view that there are grounds for classifying aphasic patients into the seven types based on patterns of impairment shown on Minnesota scores, but gives support for Schuell's later plans to revise her classification along severity lines (Schuell, 1973; revised by Sefer). Powell *et al.* (1979) examined the relationships between Schuell's seven categories of aphasia and their own four severity groups. They found a good degree of consistency between the Minnesota categories of simple aphasia, aphasia with visual involvement and mild aphasia with persisting dysfluency and their own mild group; aphasia with scattered findings and their own low-moderate category; aphasia with sensorimotor involvement and aphasia with intermittent auditory imperception with the high-moderate group and the irreversible aphasic syndrome with the severe group. Powell *et al.*'s continuum of severity coincides with Schuell's own hierarchy of severity.

Despite the fact that this analysis was unable to find statistical support for Schuell's classification, the authors emphasise that their study does not refer to the prognostic value of the classification, or the evidence that Schuell and her co-workers have put forward concerning the neurological correlates of the seven groups. Neither does it mean that classifications obtained by other means (e.g. the Boston classification) are not valid. The results of this analysis may be strongly related to the design, structure and scoring of the Minnesota.

Appraisal

The popularity of the Minnesota probably owes a great deal to its simple administration and scoring as well as its comprehensiveness and predictive power. This in turn highlights its limitations from the point of view of planning treatment. The plus-minus scoring method is insensitive to the extent that patients who appear on clinical judgement to have made progress may not show this progress on repeated testing. Against the test's comprehensiveness, the studies cited above have shown it to be highly redundant to the extent that just four subtests are sufficient to classify 87 per cent of patients. Some of the printed materials are dull, which is a criticism which can be levelled at many aphasia tests, and there appears to be no logical order in the arrangement of stimulus cards.

A more important limitation from the point of view of planning treatment however, is that the test lacks illustrative graphs and interpretative profiles to help the clinician with planning remediation, such that planning detailed treatment programmes requires time-consuming and laborious inspection of individual subtest scores. The lack of statistical treatment of raw scores does not help the clinician and unequal numbers of items within subtests makes interpretation difficult. Many clinicians prefer to convert the error scores into correct scores and compute percentages for subtests in order to make more sense of the results. A profile like the Frenchay Hospital Aphasia Assessment record (Figure 5.2) presents the patient's performance in an immediately meaningful manner. The patient's performance on re-test can be instantly compared to the initial test, deficit and retained areas

Figure 5.2: Minnesota Assessment Summary Form

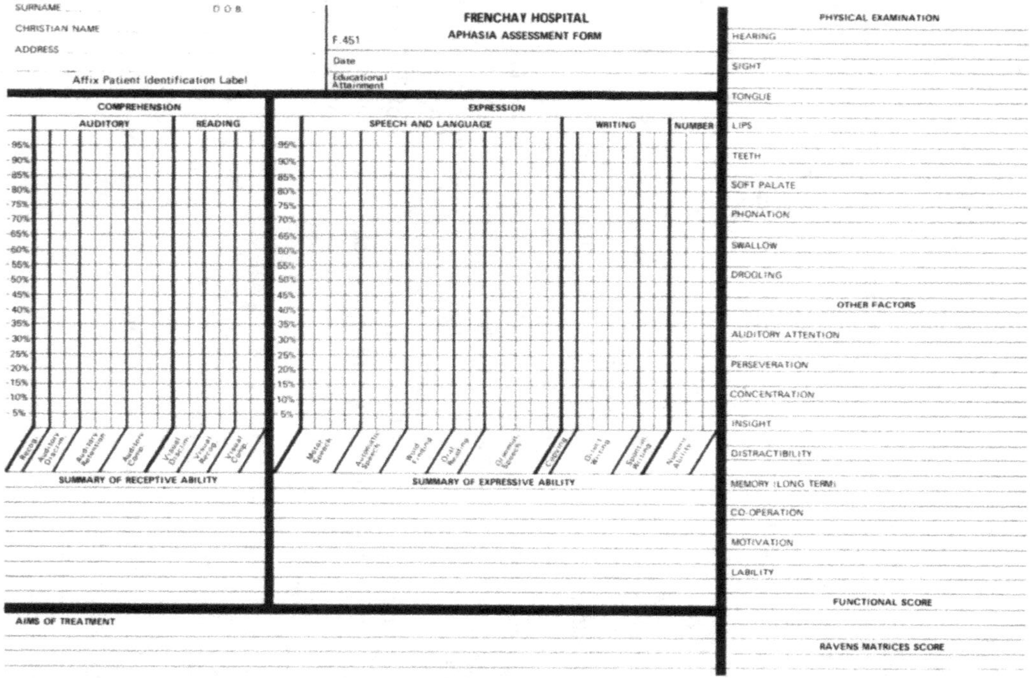

Source: Reproduced with special permission of Pam Enderby, Chief Speech Therapist, Frenchay Hospital, Bristol.

can be seen at a glance and the clinician is provided with the information required for planning treatment.

The Boston Diagnostic Aphasia Examination (Boston)

Theoretical Background

It was the intention of the authors of the Boston (Goodglass and Kaplan, 1972) to devise an assessment procedure that would diagnose the presence and type of aphasia, to aid in the localisation of cerebral damage, to measure the changes in performance on a wide range of linguistic abilities over time and to determine the deficits and retained abilities of the patient in all areas as a guide to planning treatment. As such, it was their intention to quantify and specify aphasic impairment.

In order to achieve these aims the Boston selects the most prominent behavioural characteristics of aphasia and some related disorders, then rates their presence or absence and severity relative to each other in order to diagnose the type of aphasia according to classical nomenclature. Implicit in the approach of Goodglass and Kaplan is the view that specific aphasic syndromes can be attributed to damage in specific cerebral locations and mechanisms. A fundamental premise of aphasia localisation is that observed aphasia types can be classified according to whether the patient presents with a *fluent* or a *non-fluent* aphasia, and that fluent aphasias are due to brain damage posterior to the central sulcus whereas non-fluent aphasias are caused by damage anterior to the central sulcus. This is in contrast to Schuell's (Jenkins *et al.*, 1975) uni-dimensional view of aphasia, but like Schuell, the Boston school rejects the expressive-receptive, input-output dichotomy (Goodglass, Quadfasel and Timberlake, 1964).

The Boston's multifactorial approach to the description of aphasia, which seeks to relate certain selective characteristics of aphasic behaviour to particular language centres and connecting mechanisms, delineates six major aphasic syndromes as well as a number of rarer 'pure' aphasias. The major types of aphasia that the Boston attempts to identify are Broca's aphasia, Wernicke's aphasia, conduction aphasia, anomia, transcortical motor aphasia and transcortical sensory aphasia. The *relative* prominence of the particular features which identify these major aphasia types is shown in Table 5.1, although it is emphasised that this table should be seen as a general guide only.

Table 5.1: Major Diagnostic Factors in Aphasia
Must be seen in *relation* to other factors in patient's problem.

	Broca's	Wernicke's	Anomia	Conduction	Trans-cortical Sensory	Trans-cortical Motor
Non-fluency	+	–	–	–	–	–
Repetition Difficulty	+	+	+	–	–	–
Paraphasia	–	+	–	+	+	–
Aud. Comp. Difficulty	–	+	–	–		
Naming Problems			+			
Word-finding Difficulty					+	
Reading Difficulty					+	
Writing Difficulty					+	
Parietal Involvement	–	+	+	–	+	

\+ Present
– Absent

(Adapted from Goodglass and Kaplan, 1972)

Description and Administration

The Boston examination is made up of some 27 subtests arranged into the five sections of Conversational and Expository Speech, Auditory Comprehension, Oral Expression, Understanding Written Language and Writing. The complete test package consists of just the manual *The Assessment of Aphasia and Related Disorders* (Goodglass and Kaplan, 1972) and 16 test cards. Record booklets are also available. The manual provides chapters on the background to the test including statistical analysis, the nature of aphasic deficit and descriptions of the major aphasic syndromes, the test procedure and rationale as well as supplementary language and non-language tests. The chapter on non-language tests is useful for assessing some of the apraxias and agnosias, which contribute to determining parietal lobe damage and aid in localisation.

Scoring on the Boston is predominantly plus-minus with points taken off for delay of response in some subtests, and ½ points are awarded for a cued response or partially correct response in the word discrimination subtest. A distinctive feature of the test is the qualitative emphasis given to noting the presence and severity or absence of articulatory difficulties and paraphasic errors and jargon. The scores obtained are expressed through a combination of an Aphasia Severity Rating Scale, a Rating Scale Profile of Speech Characteristics and a Z-Score Profile of Aphasia Subscores. Interpretation of the resulting patterns of deficit aid classification into the major syndromes.

Figure 5.3: Completed Aphasia Severity Rating Scale, Rating Scale Profile and Z–Score Profile from the Boston Test of a Broca's Aphasic Patient

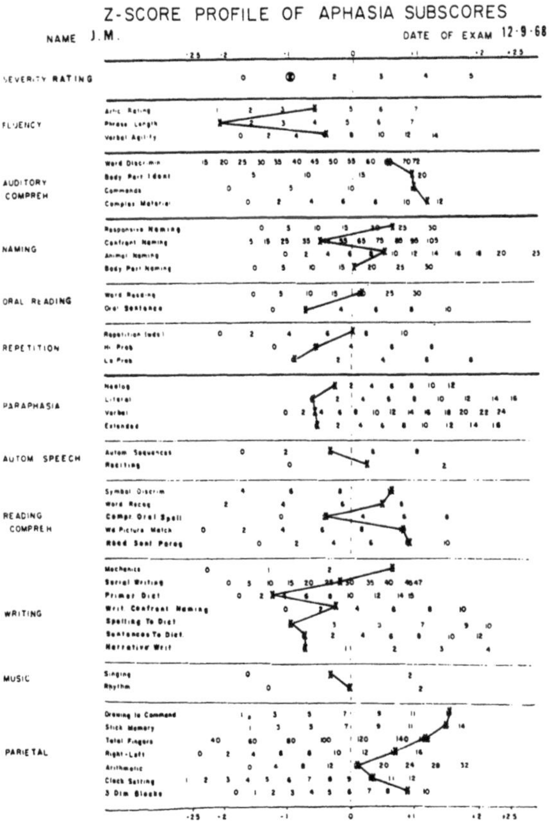

Figure 5.3: contd

Patient's Name J. M. Date of rating 2 - 26 - 70

Rated by H. G.

APHASIA SEVERITY RATING SCALE

0. No usable speech or auditory comprehension.

(1.) All communication is through fragmentary expression; great need for inference, questioning and guessing by the listener. The range of information which can be exchanged is limited, and the listener carries the burden of communication.

2. Conversation about familiar subjects is possible with help from the listener. There are frequent failures to convey the idea, but patient shares the burden of communication with the examiner.

3. The patient can discuss almost all everyday problems with little or no assistance. However, reduction of speech and/or comprehension make conversation about certain material difficult or impossible.

4. Some obvious loss of fluency in speech or facility of comprehension, without significant limitation on ideas expressed or form of expression.

5. Minimal discernible speech handicaps; patient may have subjective difficulties which are not apparent to listener.

RATING SCALE PROFILE OF SPEECH CHARACTERISTICS

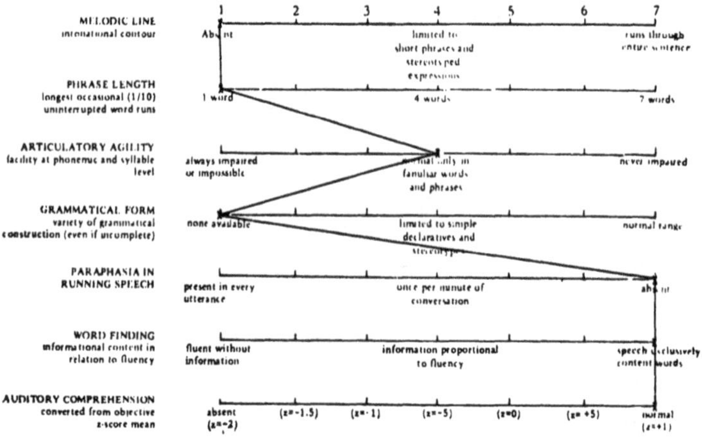

Source: Reproduced by special permission from *The Assessment of Aphasia and Related Disorders* by H. Goodglass and E. Kaplan. Copyright, 1972. Published by Lea and Febiger.

Figures 5.3 and 5.4 show the rating scales and Z-score profiles of a Broca's aphasic patient and a Wernicke's aphasic patient. It can be seen that the Rating Scale Profiles of Speech Characteristics of the two types of aphasia are in striking contrast. The patient with Broca's aphasia has difficulties with language which involve disruption of melodic line, phrase length, articulatory agility and grammatical form; whereas the patient with Wernicke's aphasia has fluent paraphasic speech which is low in information content, accompanied by an auditory comprehension deficit.

Figure 5.4: Completed Aphasia Severity Rating Scale, Rating Scale Profile and Z–Score Profile from the Boston Test of a Wernicke's Aphasic Patient

Patient's Name A. M. Date of rating 2-7-70

Rated by H. G.

APHASIA SEVERITY RATING SCALE

0. No usable speech or auditory comprehension.

(1.) All communication is through fragmentary expression; great need for inference, questioning and guessing by the listener. The range of information which can be exchanged is limited, and the listener carries the burden of communication.

2. Conversation about familiar subjects is possible with help from the listener. There are frequent failures to convey the idea, but patient shares the burden of communication with the examiner.

3. The patient can discuss almost all everyday problems with little or no assistance. However, reduction of speech and/or comprehension make conversation about certain material difficult or impossible.

4. Some obvious loss of fluency in speech or facility of comprehension, without significant limitation on ideas expressed or form of expression.

5. Minimal discernible speech handicaps; patient may have subjective difficulties which are not apparent to listener.

RATING SCALE PROFILE OF SPEECH CHARACTERISTICS

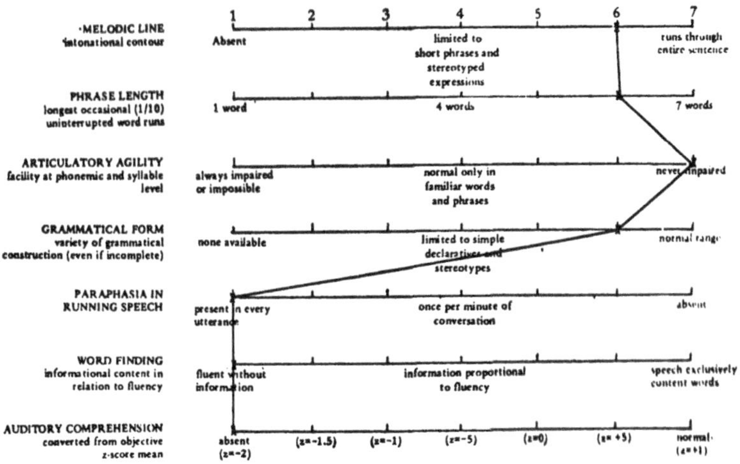

Figure 5.4: contd

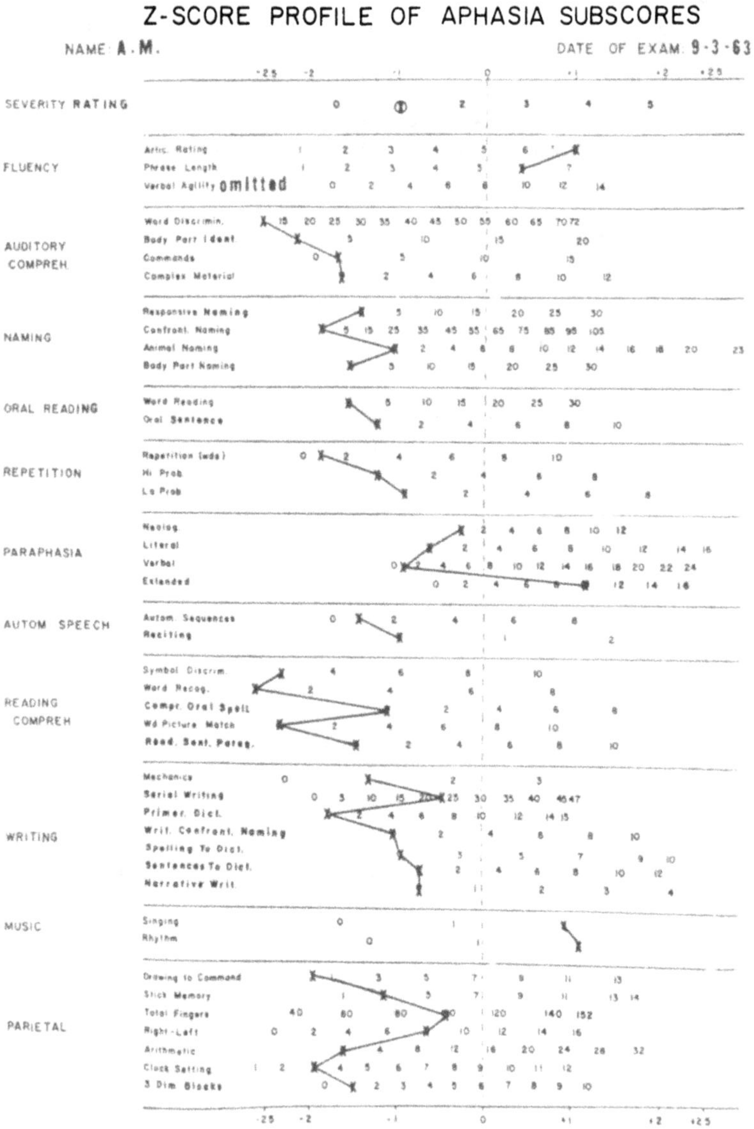

Source: Reproduced by special permission from *The Assessment of Aphasia and Related Disorders* by H. Goodglass and E. Kaplan. Copyright, 1972. Published by Lea and Febiger.

Therapeutic Implications

The usefulness of the Boston in indicating possible therapeutic strategies may be unique due to the special consideration it gives to the presence or absence and relative severity of particular aphasic characteristics. As has been discussed, special consideration is given to selective impairment of different semantic word categories, fluency, degree and type of paraphasia and auditory comprehension, as well as supplementary language and non-language tests to qualify further specific areas of deficit. The Rating Scale Profile of Speech Characteristics and Z-Score Profile provide useful guides to selection of areas for consideration for treatment. The specification of particular symptoms which contribute to a patient's individual difficulties allows the clinician to select treatment procedures for those features.

The emphasis in the structure of the test on determining the relative prominence of aphasic characteristics enables the clinician to plan remediation for those features which contribute most to the patient's problems. Detailed qualitative information on such aspects as impairment of semantic word categories enables the clinician to identify specific anomic problems for which to plan treatment, rather than adopting an unsystematic blanket approach to the remediation of 'word-finding difficulty'. Evaluation of the relative degree and type of paraphasic errors in a patient's speech provides the clinician with the necessary information required to plan therapy aimed at remediation of the most salient paraphasic problem. Changes in abilities can be determined on re-test with the Boston with improvement expressed on the test profiles and easily interpreted. The ability of the Boston to localise the underlying brain damage may not be of direct relevance to planning remediation, but will be information that may be useful to other members of the management team for making clinical decisions.

Related Research

A number of studies have been conducted to investigate the reliability of localising brain damage by reference to aphasic symptoms. Benson (1967) compared the Boston results of 50 patients classified as fluent and non-fluent and found a correlation between fluent aphasia and posterior brain damage and non-fluent aphasia and anterior brain damage, as determined by radio nuclide brain scans. Naeser and Hayward (1978) compared the Boston test results of 19 aphasic patients with computerised tomography scans and found that it was possible to determine the general site of damage by reference to the

Boston classification for most classical aphasia types. Good correlations between Boston classification and scan results were obtained for Broca's, Wernicke's conduction and transcortical motor aphasia as well as global aphasia. Other aphasia types were not included. Kertesz, Harlock and Coates (1979) in a similar study have confirmed that anomic aphasia evolves from Broca's and Wernicke's aphasia, rather than from a separate cerebral lesion. These results tend to confirm the view that general sites of lesions can be determined for some types of aphasia. Kerschensteiner, Poeck and Brunner (1972) have criticised this kind of study, arguing that aphasia must be classified in terms of language behaviour alone and they suggest that the terms anterior-posterior be discarded with reference to the fluent and non-fluent types of aphasia.

A number of investigations have sought to confirm the importance of the behavioural characteristics which the Boston attempts to measure (see Goodglass, 1978, for a collection of some of the main studies). The fluency and non-fluency distinction originally proposed by Howes and Geschwind (Howes and Geschwind, 1964; Howes, 1964; Geschwind, 1966) was the subject of a study by Kerschensteiner *et al.* (1972). They conducted a cluster-analysis of the spontaneous speech of 47 unselected aphasic subjects which indicated that the fluency and non-fluency distinction 'reflects naturally occurring differences in language behaviour' (p. 245). They looked at ten language variables and found that the most discriminating for classification into fluent and non-fluent were prosody, rate of speaking, phrase length and pauses. Goodglass, Quadfasel and Timberlake (1964) used the Aphasia Severity Rating Scale and the Rating Scale Profile of Speech Characteristics of the Boston to rate the performances of 53 aphasic subjects on the Conversational and Expository Speech and the Auditory Comprehension sections of the test. They found that phrase length, that is, the length of uninterrupted word sequences, distinguished sharply between Broca's patients on the one hand, and Wernicke's patients on the other.

The Boston contains four subtests of naming; responsive naming, visual confrontation naming – including objects, letters, geometric forms, numbers and colours, a subtest for body-part naming and another for animal naming. Support for this exhaustive assessment of naming comes from Goodglass, Klein, Carey and Jones (1966) who tested a group of Broca's, Wernicke's and anomic aphasic subjects (135 in all) on a variety of naming tasks and found that naming objects was the most difficult for all three classes of subjects, but one of the easiest to comprehend. Letters, on the other hand, were the easiest to name, but the hardest to comprehend. Wernicke's patients had particular difficulties with body-part comprehension and Wernicke's and anomic subjects had relatively good letter naming and poor object naming. No significant differences were found in the naming ability of Broca's aphasics for the various semantic classes.

Factor analysis has been carried out twice on the Boston and reported in Goodglass and Kaplan (1972). A comparison of both analyses revealed a first factor related to reading and writing tasks and a second factor related to performance on the parietal lobe battery of the test. Fluency and articulatory agility, as well as repetition and recitation, were represented on a third factor, and a fourth factor represented by auditory comprehension and paraphasia emerged, which was interpreted as a 'Wernicke's aphasia' factor. An 'anomic' factor did not emerge and Goodglass and Kaplan state that this is due to the masking effect of severity of aphasia and the limitations of factor analysis. Goodglass and Kaplan were more selective in their choice of subjects for these analyses than Schuell, Jenkins and Carroll (1962) were for their factor analysis of the Minnesota test, and they defend the selective approach as necessary to demonstrate the independence of factors. They chose subjects who had symptoms in *relative* isolation and they point out that 'although this smacks of circular reasoning and data manipulation, it has more to recommend it than the indiscriminating accumulation of consecutive cases without concern for the make up of the population' (p. 15). They were also able to report good reliability co-efficients for the subtests of the battery indicating good internal consistency within subtests.

Appraisal

The scoring of the Boston requires more attention and consideration to details of the patient's responses than the Minnesota, but this should not be seen as a disadvantage. The more detail about the patient's disabilities clinicians have at their disposal, the better able they are to plan appropriate and effective treatment. Goodglass and his associates (Goodglass, Quadfasel and Timberlake, 1964) acknowledge that the determination of aphasia type with the Boston test is achieved more by subjective assessment of the patient's spontaneous speech during the first section (Conversational and Expository Speech) than by reference to the objective scores of the rest of the battery. This subjective rating of the first six features in the Rating Scale Profile of Speech Characteristics, together with a rating of auditory comprehension taken from objective scores, is sufficient to classify type of aphasia. This would suggest that from a diagnostic standpoint much of the battery may be redundant. The problem is, as Goodglass *et al.* (1964) have pointed out, that it is very difficult to measure critical variables, like phrase length, in a quantitative manner without resorting to rating scales. The Minnesota also depends in part on rating the severity of twelve features in its Diagnostic Scale, although most of the information on severity necessary to rate those twelve features is gained through objective scores.

The therapeutic value of the Boston lies in its ability to differentiate aphasic types, indicate the relative severity of particular characteristics of the patient's problem and provide special consideration for particular symptoms. The test is comprehensive, although like in the Minnesota gesture and pantomime are not assessed. This seems strange, especially as Goodglass and Kaplan (1963) are themselves responsible for one of the major studies on the subject, but they were probably not included because assessment of gesture and pantomime does not help a great deal in determining aphasia type. Stimulus materials are minimal and the test is very portable, although the size and quality of the illustrations may leave something to be desired. The methods chosen for expressing the results of the test provide much information for the clinician concerned with planning treatment, although much of this qualitative data may actually be redundant for diagnosis of type of aphasia.

The Porch Index of Communicative Ability

Theoretical Background

The PICA (Porch, 1967) was developed to answer a need in speech pathology for an assessment of aphasia that was sensitive to minimal changes in performance, would aid in the prediction of recovery, was reliable and objective and independent of particular theoretical explanations of aphasic breakdown. Porch (1971) employs the notion of a ranked communication task continuum as a basic framework for quantitative and qualitative measurement, with more difficult and complex tasks at one end and easier and more automatic tasks at the other. For Porch (1971) 'the purpose of testing is to locate the point on the continuum at which the patient is functioning' (p. 74).

The unique features of the PICA are not its theoretical rationale or choice of test items, but its *multidimensional scoring system* and highly *formal administration*, which were designed to increase the sensitivity of aphasia testing. Five dimensions are used to describe responses on the PICA which are considered to encompass most of the important features observable in aphasia. The five descriptive dimensions are accuracy, responsiveness, completeness, promptness and efficiency. Porch (1971) describes five basic types of profile that emerge on testing with PICA. These are: aphasia without complications; aphasia with verbal formulation or expression problems due to either apraxia, dysarthria or inadequate verbal monitoring; aphasia complicated by illiteracy; patterns indicative of bilateral brain damage; aberrant patterns which indicate problems which are not aphasic in nature.

Description and Administration

The PICA consists of 18 subtests each containing ten assessment tasks which claim to measure communicative abilities in three modalities (four verbal, eight gestural, six graphic). The patient is required to respond to a variety of commands centred around ten test objects (pen, pencil, quarter/ten pence-piece, cigarette, box of matches, knife, fork, key, comb, toothbrush) which were chosen because they are common everyday items to both sexes, are instantly recognisable and may all be manipulated in some way by hand. The 18 subtests of the PICA are arranged in decreasing order of difficulty because it was felt that this would have the effect of encouraging the patient who would find that his performance was improving as he went through the test rather than deteriorating. This is in contrast to the strategy employed in the other clinical batteries described in this chapter, where an increasing hierarchy of difficulty is utilised.

The multidimensional scoring scale of the PICA was designed to provide the tester with a range of scores from 1 to 16 to award for a given response to an item, which would describe the response numerically in terms of the five descriptive dimensions referred to above. On a given test task a patient would score 16 (Complex) for a response which is accurate, responsive, complex, immediate and elaborative. A score of 15 (Complete) is assigned to a response which is accurate, responsive, complete and immediate, and a score of 14 (Distorted) for an accurate, responsive, complete response which is distorted. A response which is complete in every way, but delayed, is given a score of 13 (Complete-Delayed) whereas a response which is incomplete is awarded 12 (Incomplete). The patient earns 11 (Incomplete-Delayed) if his response is both incomplete and delayed and 10 (Corrected) if he corrects a previously incorrect response without intervening variables. If the tester needs to provide a repetition of the test command and the response is correct in terms of the five dimensions, the patient scores 9 (Repetition), and if a cue is necessary to produce a response 8 (Cued) is scored. A response which is inaccurate but clearly related to the required response is given a score of 7 (Related) and an inaccurate response is awarded 6 (Error). An intelligible but incorrect and unrelated response is given 5 (Intelligible), but an unintelligible response scores 4 (Unintelligible) provided it can be differentiated from other responses. A score of 3 (Minimal) is earned for a response which is incomprehensible and cannot be differentiated from other responses. If the patient gives no response but at least attends to the test item, he is given a score of 2 (Attention), and even if the patient shows no awareness whatever of the test item he scores 1 (No Response).

It can be seen that the multidimensional scoring system attempts to quantify and specify any possible response in numerical terms, which, it is claimed, enables detailed description of impairment and the detection of minute changes in communicative performance on re-test.

The scores obtained on each item in a given subtest are added up and the mean is computed by dividing by ten (the number of items in each subtest) to give a Subtest Mean. An Overall Score can be calculated by averaging all 18 Subtest Means. Porch (1971) suggests that the Overall Score 'is the best single index of the patient's general communicative ability. Its simplest interpretation is that of placing the patient's performance on the battery at a particular point on a sixteen-step scale of adequacy with 1.00 being the least adequate performance and 16 being the most adequate' (p. 70). Means can also be separately calculated for the three modalities of the test and expressed graphically on the Modality Response Summary (Figure 5.5) and Subtest Means can also be plotted on the Ranked Response Summary (Figure 5.6). The Modality Response means give an indication of the patient's relative abilities in each of the three modalities, and according to Porch (1971) an unselected sample of aphasic patients will produce mean gestural levels of about 12.00, verbal of about 10.00 and graphic of about 8.00. In the Ranked Response Summary the subtests are arranged according to difficulty from Test A (most difficult) to Test XI (least difficult). The diagonal line represents the mean score on each subtest for a sample of 190 aphasic patients, and it can be seen that these mean scores range from about 6.00 for subtest A to 14.00 for subtest XI.

Therapeutic Implications

According to Porch (1971) 'the clinician has at his disposal 180 descriptions of how the patient performs in a test situation' (p. 102). The PICA manual (Porch, 1971) gives guidance to interpretation and analysis which helps provide a basis for prognosis and treatment. The highest scores obtained by a patient on a given subtest, for instance, can be interpreted as *a potential level of performance* on that task. With improvement the patient should be able to achieve this score for all the items in that particular subtest. As a general rule, the more higher scores the patient achieves on a given subtest, as well as the greater variety of scores, the better the patient's chances of improvement on that subtest.

Figure 5.5: Modality Response Summary of the PICA

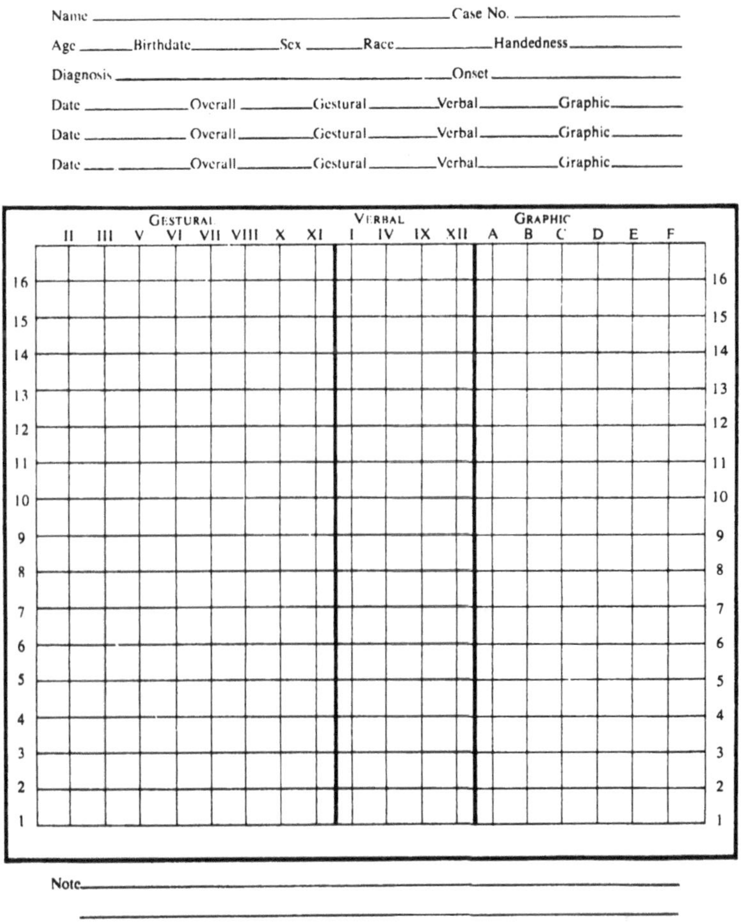

Source: Reproduced by special permission from *The Porch Index of Communicative Ability* by B. Porch, PhD. Copyright 1967 and 1971. Published by Consulting Psychologists Press Inc.

Figure 5.6: Ranked Response Summary of the PICA

Name ________________ Case No. ________________

Age ____ Birthdate ____ Sex ____ Race ____ Handedness ____

Diagnosis ________________ Onset ________________

Date ____ Overall ____ Gestural ____ Verbal ____ Graphic ____

Date ____ Overall ____ Gestural ____ Verbal ____ Graphic ____

Date ____ Overall ____ Gestural ____ Verbal ____ Graphic ____

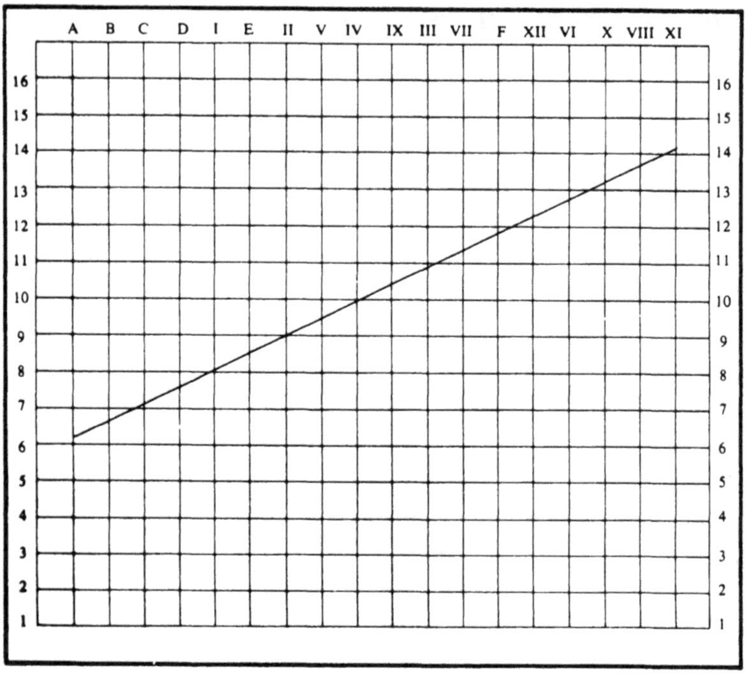

Note ________________________________

Source: Reproduced by special permission from *The Porch Index of Communicative Ability* by B. Porch, PhD. Copyright 1967 and 1971. Published by Consulting Psychologists Press Inc.

The Subtest Means can be seen as an indication of the patient's ability on specific test tasks in terms of the five dimensions, and inspection of actual subtest scores may provide additional information regarding the patient's pattern of impairment. For instance, if the score 9 (Repetition) appears frequently at the beginning of subtests, it would indicate that the patient has difficulty with auditory comprehension to the extent that he requires repetition of commands.

The notion of the ranked communication task continuum is employed by Porch (1971) as a basis for planning therapy where treatment is directed 'at those tasks and skills which are adjacent to the most difficult tasks at which the patient has complete success; that is, tasks at which he has no deficit in any of the five dimensions of response' (p. 74). Predictable recovery patterns are observable on the PICA according to Porch, in so far as it is reasonable to assume that with improvement and on re-test the patient will move up the task continuum in a predictable way, either gradually or in several large steps.

A further feature of PICA analysis is the Aphasia Recovery Curve (Figure 5.7) which, it is claimed, is 'invaluable as a sensitive indicant of the effects of treatment, time, surgery, or other variables' (Porch, 1971, p. 111). The clinician first takes the patient's overall score and finds the Overall Percentile (O) by reference to the relevant table in the manual. The next step is to find the nine highest subtest scores from the 18, compute the mean, and look up the Nine-High Percentile (H) in the manual. The same is done for the nine lowest subtest scores which gives the Nine-Low Percentile (L). The clinician then simply plots these three percentiles – the Overall (O), the Nine-High (H) and the Nine-Low (L), on the Aphasia Recovery Curve sheet as illustrated in Figure 5.7. A large High-Low gap would indicate much room for improvement, whereas a non-existent gap suggests that the patient has achieved his maximum recovery provided his condition has stabilised. One of the aims of treatment is to erase this gap. Further prediction can be made with the so-called HOAP (High-Overall Prediction) Method. This involves simply finding the Overall percentile which is closest to the patient's overall percentile in the data provided in the manual at one month post-onset, and then finding the high score level which is most similar to the patient's overall score. This *high* score can be seen as an indication of the sort of Overall score that the patient should achieve at six months post-onset.

Figure 5.7: Aphasia Recovery Curve of the PICA

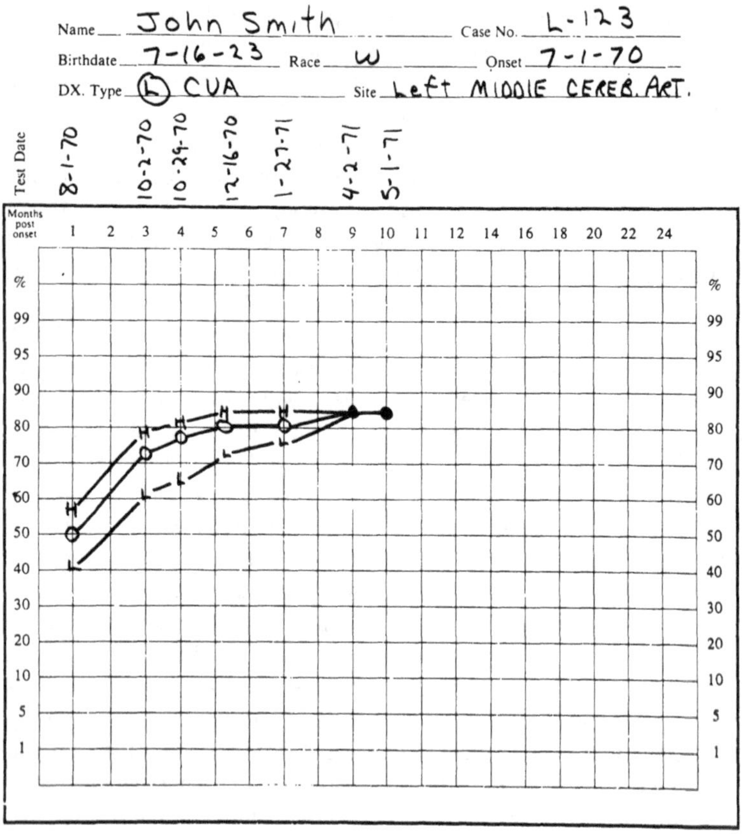

Souce: Reproduced by special permission from *The Porch Index of Communicative Ability* by B. Porch, PhD. Copyright, 1967 and 1971. Published by Consulting Psychologists Press Inc.

Related Research

Hanson and Cicciarelli (1978) looked at the time, amount and pattern of change in the PICA scores of 13 aphasic patients and found that the degree of recovery as well as the level of completeness of recovery was related to the level of severity on initial assessment. Patients with the highest overall scores improved the most, although patients with low overall scores did show significant positive change. Peak improvement was reached within 8.63 months post-onset for the group as a whole. A study by Porch, Collins, Wertz and Friden (1980) examined the test and re-test PICA scores of 144 subjects and found that it was statistically possible to predict recovery in aphasia, that the most significant predictor was the Gestural Mean and that a patient's communicative performance may be more important for prediction than age.

DiSimoni, Keith, Holt and Darley (1975) have suggested that there are a number of reasons for shortening the PICA, not least because the test takes from sixty to ninety minutes to administer. This suggestion is made despite Porch's claim that some reliability might be lost by shortening the test. DiSimoni *et al.* point out that redundancy would be indicated in the PICA by the consistently high correlations reported by Porch between subtests, and they subjected the PICA scores of 222 subjects to stepwise regression analysis. Their results indicated that just four subtest mean scores could predict overall scores successfully. They were concerned to point out that their analysis does not refer to the reliability of a short version or to the prognostic value of the PICA. Phillips and Halpin (1978) examined the reliability of two shortened versions of the PICA which they assessed to be only slightly lower than the full version. They also found basically identical means and standard deviations for subtest, modality and overall scores between the two short versions and the long version. Also, the Modality Response Summary, Ranked Response Summary and other analyses can be done in the same way as for the full length version. The two short versions were determined by reducing each subtest to five commands associated with five test objects rather than the ten objects in the full length version. A further reason for eliminating some of the test objects is one of hygiene where Phillips and Halpin consider that the toothbrush, cigarette, fork and comb are often used too literally by patients.

Clark, Crockett and Klonoff's (1979a; 1979b) factor analysis of the PICA revealed that five dimensions of language ability accounted for 90 per cent of the variance of the subtests. These factors were fluency, graphic expression, gestural demonstration of comprehension, gesturing the function of an object and graphic-copying. Clark *et al.* (1979b) suggest that the PICA should be modified to measure these five dimensions. Their analysis confirmed the notion of an overall score which reflects a general communicative competence, but rejected Porch's notion of a gestural modality as defined and tested by the PICA. Moreover, Subtest F (graphic-copying) is loaded with the gestural factor and they therefore suggest that it should be omitted from calculations of graphic ability.

Appraisal

Martin (1977) has raised a number of questions concerning the PICA. He points out that there are cases where the multidimensional scoring system fails to capture details of a patient's response and that the test ignores non-verbal aspects of communication. Furthermore, the PICA does not directly assess comprehension – a point also noted by Boone (1972), and the rigid administration instructions of the test do not allow the examiner to intervene and make a clear determination of the comprehension level of the patient. Martin criticises Porch's insistence on forcing tests like the reading tests (5 and 7) into the *gestural* modality simply because the cards with the printed instructions must be *placed* in certain positions by the patient. Martin (1977) comments that 'the nature of the response, which was so highly prized in the rationale for the scoring system, has now been distorted beyond retrieval by ignoring the nature of the task for the sake of "modality" scoring' (p. 554). Some support for this criticism has been supplied by Clark *et al.*'s (1979a) factor analysis which showed that the so-called gestural subtests did not load 'cleanly', which suggests that they do not provide a good measure of gestural ability.

Martin also raises questions concerning the statistical treatment of subtest scores with the PICA. He refers to an article by Silverman (1974) who showed that a given subtest mean score can numerically represent a response that did not actually occur during the subtest. Martin further states that two separate kinds of task response (e.g. refusing to carry out a task and an automatic speech response) can both be awarded a score of 5, implying numerical equivalence for both behaviours which will be reflected in the statistical treatment of scores. Martin considers the lack of theoretical depth to the PICA to be a disadvantage and questions its reliability as a test of aphasia.

A high level augmentation to the PICA is under development which contains nine new subtests described as advanced. The subtests include two for auditory comprehension, two for drawing, two for reading, one gestural and two verbal. Some of these items have no doubt been included to answer some of the criticisms levelled at the PICA and may serve to extend the validity of the battery. The new gestural subtest, for instance, requires the patient to demonstrate the function of the objects through pantomime without actually using the objects, and may therefore be a more genuine test of non-verbal communicative abilities. The new reading tests are not subsumed under the 'gestural' modality and the auditory comprehension tests have been included so that this aspect of language can be directly assessed.

The PICA claims to be able to describe in sensitive numerical detail the communicative competence of the patient and should consequently provide the clinician with a mass of information about the patient's abilities at the time of testing, predictive information on the kind of recovery pattern the patient will follow and minute changes in abilities on retest. The foregoing discussion has shown that there are certain inconsistencies in the scoring system of the PICA. These may affect some of the claims of the test and it should not be seen as an all-powerful tool without defects, but as a potentially excellent assessment procedure from the clinician's point of view, requiring on-going research and development to highlight its strengths and weaknesses. Much effort has gone into the design of the PICA to systematise scoring, and into analysis and interpretation of scores to help the clinician in making decisions concerning treatment. The Modality Response Summary presents a visual representation of the relative contribution of separate modality difficulties to the patient's problems, although the remarks noted above should be borne in mind in evaluation of the 'gestural' modality. The Ranked Response Summary provides the same visual presentation of subtest means to aid placement of the patient on the ranked communication task continuum, and reference to scores for individual items can reveal the type and frequency of responses to particular test items. The test in its standard form does not directly assess comprehension and, due to its systematic nature, no evaluation of spontaneous speech is included.

In defence of the PICA's lack of theoretical depth, it must be said that the PICA was never designed to make a contribution to our understanding of the nature of aphasia *per se*, but to be a detailed measuring technique which would provide more information to aid the clinician in determining likely recovery patterns for patients, and to make the most detailed possible statement of the patient's abilities and deficits to help in planning treatment to maximise that recovery.

Functional Communication Profile (FCP)

Theoretical Background

Taylor-Sarno (Taylor-Sarno, 1969; Taylor, 1965) argues that standard aphasia tests give a false impression of the patient's communicative abilities because they assess *clinical* performance without reference to a patient's abilities to cope with real life situations involving communication. In other words, there is no automatic and necessary correlation between an individual's scores on a clinical aphasia battery and *functional* communicative capabilities. The FCP aims to assess the patient's functional communicative abilities.

Taylor (1965) defines a measure of language use as functional 'when the conditions or stimuli used are informal and they sample language usage without task presentation' (p. 102). As an example of the two types of performance Taylor cites the act of patients writing their name to command in the clinic and signing a cheque in a bank: the former is a clinical and the latter a functional performance. Standard batteries assess clinical performance and provide the clinician with few indications as to the patient's ability to compensate for reduced linguistic skills in natural and informal communicative situations. Taylor points out that most clinical tests do not take account of a patient's compensatory use of gesture and other paralinguistic aspects of communication, and often penalise slow, linguistically inaccurate or inconsistent responses. Furthermore, the severely and minimally impaired are unassessable on some batteries. Many severe patients are unable even to attempt some clinical tests, whereas others are often insensitive to minimal problems.

The FCP makes no reference to any typology of aphasia or to diagnostic categories, and has no specific theoretical basis, except its distinction between 'clinical' and 'functional' notions of aphasia assessment.

Description and Administration

The FCP simply consists of a form which contains a list of 45 common communicative functions of everyday life. These 45 language functions are arranged into the five categories of movement (e.g. ability to indicate 'yes' and 'no'), speaking (e.g. saying phrases), understanding (e.g. recognition of names of familiar objects), reading (e.g. reading street signs) and other (e.g. handling money, time orientation). These categories were established on the basis of a factor analysis carried out on the items included (Taylor, 1965). Each of the 45 communicative behaviours is assessed by the clinician during informal conversational interaction and rated on an eight point scale which ranges from 'normal' (the patient performs the task exactly as he did pre-morbidly) to very poor. These ratings can then be converted to percentages for each of the five categories of activity and an Overall Score can be obtained. An Overall Score of 69 per cent for example, means that patients' overall functional communicative ability is rated at 69 per cent of their pre-morbid ability.

Rating on the FCP should be obtained from informal everyday life and based on first-hand observation where possible. A non-structured interview is suggested, although some items cannot be observed in a quasi-natural setting, like writing to dictation, oral movements and copying ability. Ratings for these items are taken from clinical tasks. Direct questioning is necessary to rate items like watching television and films, as well as information gained second-hand from relatives and friends.

It is suggested that the clinician does not take notes during the interview, but completes the form immediately after the informal exchange which should take between 15 and 30 minutes. Apart from these general guidelines there is no formal administrative script for the tester to follow. It is suggested that re-assessment should be done, at least, on a monthly basis (Taylor-Sarno, 1969).

Related Research

A shortened version of the FCP has been developed (Edwards, Ellams and Thompson, 1976; Walker and Williams, 1980) using a five point rating scale of just 20 functional language skills. Positive inter-tester reliability correlation co-efficients of over 0.9 for each section were established for two testers on 6 subjects, although the two testers had considerable preliminary discussion. Edwards *et al.* (1976) compared the revised FCP scores with Minnesota scores of 62 aphasic subjects and observed a positive correlation of above 0.9 which suggests that this version of the FCP is a valid measure.

Anderson, Bouveston and Greenberg (1971) observed a good relationship between full FCP scores and Minnesota scores, but Needham and Swisher (1972) tested 25 subjects and found that when scores on the understanding section of the FCP, an aphasia battery and the Token Test were compared, there was no correlation between FCP scores and the combined Token Test and battery scores. Further analysis suggested that the possible reason for the discrepancies between the 'clinical' tests and the FCP could be due to a degree of subjectivity on the part of the examiner in rating the FCP. They suggested that the tester could have been influenced by knowledge that the patient had brain damage which might influence rating on the higher level items. Furthermore, the five subjects in the study with scores of 10 per cent lower than the clinical tests presented with some verbal apraxia as well as aphasia. They conclude that the lack of similarity between comprehension scores of the FCP and the clinical tests was due mainly to the presence of verbal apraxia or dysarthria influencing the testers' rating of performance. Consequently, such patients may be incorrectly rated on the FCP understanding section.

Egolf and Chester (1977) conducted a study in which they were concerned to compare the verbal performance of aphasic patients in the speech therapy clinic with performance in other departments of a rehabilitation centre, using the observations of professional workers other than speech therapists. Their general conclusions support Anderson *et al.* (1971) in so far as they found that there was variability between groups of informants in the reliability of their observations, especially in estimations of comprehension. Other studies (Helmick, Watamori and Palmer, 1976; Flowers, Beukelman, Bottorf and Kelley, 1979) which have looked at relatives' understanding of the deficits of aphasic patients imply that relatives should not be considered good judges of communicative abilities. However, Holland (1977) has criticised the study of Helmick *et al.* on the grounds that scores from the PICA (a clinical battery), which were used to establish the *objective* criterion, cannot be meaningfully compared to the naturalistic evaluations of the patient's relatives.

These points are significant for interpretation of FCP scores as it is suggested by Taylor-Sarno (1969) that the profile should not be used by clinicians with small case-loads and little experience with aphasic patients. Taylor and Sands (1965) examined the inter-rater reliability of the FCP as well as test-retest and found that inter-rater reliability correlations ranged from +0.87 to +0.95 and test-retest reliability was also reported to be high. It therefore appears that rating on the FCP can be influenced by subjectivity to some degree and is a direct reflection of the rater's experience and knowledge. It is the case, however, that scoring on any test must be influenced to some extent by the experience and knowledge of the tester.

Therapeutic Implications

The FCP makes no reference to symptomological or diagnostic categories and was not intended to be a substitute for comprehensive assessment of linguistic skills. It gives no suggestions or directions to the clinician for treatment. From the point of view of rehabilitation the value of the FCP is its emphasis on functional abilities, its power to measure the patient's capacity to cope in real life situations with reduced communicative skills. Heilporn (1978) reminds the clinician that 'the ultimate aim of rehabilitation is the restoration of the disabled to participation in the social and vocational activities of a normal life, however severe the patient's handicaps' (p. 22).

The FCP should have particular relevance where vocational and social considerations are concerned. To do a particular job of work a certain functional level of communication is required which may be independent to some degree of clinical levels of ability as determined by standard aphasia tests. Again, a functional level of communicative competence is essential to the maintainance and development of human relationships, as well as other psychosocial aspects of rehabilitation for aphasic patients. It is probably the case that psychosocial adjustment to aphasic handicap is more dependent upon good functional recovery than good linguistic recovery, although research is required to determine what relationships exist between functional communicative abilities and psychosocial adjustment.

The assessment of everyday functional abilities raises the question of a form of therapy which is directed more at improving functional abilities than clinical ones. Prinz (1980) has confirmed that aphasic patients, irrespective of severity of linguistic impairment, are capable of employing pragmatic strategies to express their needs. Even global aphasic patients will utilise gesture and contextual information in order to achieve communicative success. The implication of this work is that more emphasis should be placed on providing opportunities for the patient to apply these strategies in everyday socio-communicative activities.

Group treatment approaches to therapy (Blackman, 1950; Aronson, Shatin and Cook, 1956; Fawcus, 1964) may be considered to be intermediate in some respects between a formal clinical treatment environment and a naturalistic one, where many of the normal everyday socio-communicative activities that people experience can be simulated. FCP assessment may be a more useful indicator of whether a patient should be assigned to a group and a measure of progress attained in functional abilities in the group.

Although the profile was not developed to classify aphasic performance according to typology, it is claimed that it will highlight specific difficulties. A patient with verbal apraxia, for instance, will produce a profile that shows an imbalance between scores on the understanding section compared to the other four sections. Similarly, a profile which shows lower than normal scores in all sections except the 'other' category reflects non-aphasic impairment due to disordered memory, perception and/or orientation.

Appraisal

Clinical experience tends to support the clinical/functional dichotomy in so far as a patient who performs badly on clinical assessment can often be seen to cope relatively well in communicative situations, making maximum use of every mode of communication at his disposal. The patient who does well on testing but never quite maximises his potential for one reason or another is also a not uncommon phenomenon in the clinic.

An attractive and important feature of the FCP is that the patient is his or her own norm in so far as functional abilities are compared to pre-morbid abilities and not to average normal performances or average aphasic performances. We are often guilty in our assessments and in our therapeutic dealings with patients of comparing individuals with averages rather than trying to see the patient's deficits and abilities, and progress or lack of progress, as the patient sees them. Even so, determining pre-morbid abilities must be to some extent approximate. For the clinician who recognises the importance of the functional aspects of therapy, the FCP is probably the best tool available at the present time to assess communicative effectiveness in daily life. Clearly there are limitations to the FCP's usefulness in suggesting specific areas of deficit for which treatment might be planned and probably the best it can do is highlight deficits in the broad areas of movement, speaking, understanding and reading. Further clinical testing will be required in order to plan therapy for specific deficits. The FCP has predictive value at least in so far as higher overall scores indicate a better prognosis than low overall scores, and the test is brief with a minimum of statistical analysis, requires no special apparatus, can assess the very mild and the very severe and there is no danger of a learning effect on retest.

The Token Test (TT) and Reporter's Test (RT)

Theoretical Background, Description and Administration

The Token Test (De Renzi and Vignolo, 1962; De Renzi and Faglioni, 1978) and the more recent expressive version of the Token Test – the Reporter's Test (De Renzi and Ferrari, 1978) – is described and discussed as a potential battery for the detection and description of aphasic impairment with special emphasis upon higher level comprehension and expression deficit. This refers to the level of comprehension and expression deficit which may be missed or only partially indicated by standard test batteries.

The original 1962 version of the TT was developed to answer a need for a sensitive test of comprehension as conventional aphasia batteries often fail to reveal mild comprehension loss. The originators wanted to design a test which assessed *only* the comprehension of language without taxing memory or intellectual ability. The authors consider that a sensitive test for receptive disturbance should have short instructions that could be easily memorised and were intellectually easy but linguistically difficult. Furthermore, the instructions should be worded in such a way that they contained no redundant elements which would aid comprehension, and it was only possible to carry out the commands successfully by comprehending every element.

The resulting TT consists of 20 coloured tokens laid out in front of the patient which are either circles or rectangles, large or small, and either red, green, blue, yellow or white. Redundancy is avoided because in order to identify a token it is necessary to comprehend its size, colour and shape. There are 61 instructions to the test which are arranged in five parts which become progressively more difficult as the assessment proceeds. The instructions start with simple commands like 'Pick up the yellow rectangle' and 'Pick up the white circle' and progress to 'Except for the green one, touch the circles' and 'Before touching the yellow circle, pick up the red rectangle'. The test takes from twenty to thirty minutes to administer and it is necessary to eliminate possible visual agnosia and visual-field defects before testing. Tokens are usually made from coloured plastic or card according to the specifications in De Renzi and Vignolo (1962).

In their original study the authors tested thirteen 'motor' aphasic subjects and six 'sensory' aphasic subjects who had made good recoveries and most of whom had never presented with any difficulties of comprehension. Definite impairment of comprehension was detected by the TT, demonstrating that they had developed a test of auditory comprehension that was extremely sensitive.

A number of revised and shortened versions of the test have been used in experimental studies to examine various aspects of comprehension in aphasia (Boller and Vignolo, 1966; Spreen and Benton, 1969; Peock and Hartje, 1979; Lesser, 1979) but the version to be considered here in detail is the De Renzi and Faglioni (1978) revision. In this version the number of test commands has been reduced to 36, with the original Parts I to IV having four instructions each and the original Part V having thirteen. A new easier section having seven commands has been included at the beginning of the test to widen its assessment capacity to include patients with more severe receptive deficits, as the more severe patients tend not to score anything on the original TT. In this new initial section, the patient is required to comprehend only one word (e.g. 'Touch the *circle*'; 'Touch the *green* one'). Squares are used instead of rectangles due to the higher frequency of the word 'square', and black tokens instead of blue originals due to the possibility of confusion between green and blue. The shortened and revised TT was administered to an unselected group of 200 aphasic subjects and a 215 subject control group (De Renzi and Faglioni, 1978).

The scores are adjusted by adding and subtracting points according to the number of years the patient has spent in schooling. A score of below 29 (the *cutting score*), from a possible maximum of 36, constitutes a pathological performance on the test, and a score above the cutting score is considered a non-aphasic performance. However, 5 per cent of non-aphasic patients are expected to achieve scores of less than 29. Aphasic scores in this study ranged from 0-33 with 7 per cent of aphasic patients achieving scores above the cutting score of 29. Therefore, the conclusion must be that some 5 per cent of non-aphasic patients and about 7 per cent of aphasic patients will be mis-diagnosed. These figures compare very well with most standard aphasia tests. A Sentence Comprehension Test was administered to 106 of the aphasic subjects, as well as the TT, which was able to detect comprehension impairment in only 60 per cent compared to the 93 per cent hit rate of the TT.

The authors suggest that, as a rough guide, non-fluent patients who score below 17 can be considered to have global aphasia and non-fluent patients with scores above 17 can be considered to be Broca's aphasics. A five-point comprehension impairment severity scale is included by the authors which designates a score of 0-8 as very severe; 9-16 as severe; 17-24 as moderate; 25-28 as mild and 29-36 as a normal performance. This shortened version takes from ten to fifteen minutes to complete.

An ingenious expressive version of the TT – the Reporter's Test – has been reported recently (De Renzi and Ferrari, 1978) which is administered following the completion of the revised TT. This is done in order to familiarise the patient with the materials and procedure. The patient is then told that the examiner is going to manipulate the tokens in certain ways and he (the patient) must imagine a third person sitting next to him who cannot see what the examiner is doing. The patient is then told to describe what the examiner does with the tokens as carefully as possible, and in as much detail as possible, so that the third fictitious person can repeat exactly the same manipulations with another set of tokens. De Renzi and Ferrari were concerned to devise a test of expressive ability that would require the patient to produce complete non-redundant sentences. Connected speech is usually encouraged in an aphasia assessment by picture description as in the Minnesota and Boston tests or open-ended conversation as in the Boston 'but this procedure leaves the examiner without a precise standard of references to which to compare the patient's verbal behaviour' (De Renzi and Ferrari, 1978, p. 280). The RT does not allow for alternative verbal descriptions and entails the obligatory use of certain elements of speech, although the authors acknowledge that a limited vocabulary is involved in describing the actions of the TT.

The RT consists of 26 commands taken from the short TT and arranged in five parts. Scoring is of two types – plus-minus and weighted. The maximum plus-minus score is 26 and the weighted score range is 0-60. The Reporter's Test was administered to a control group of 70 normal subjects, 60 aphasic subjects selected for absence of severe expressive impairment, 20 non-aphasic left hemisphere-damaged subjects and 20 non-aphasic right hemisphere-damaged patients (De Renzi and Ferrari, 1978). As with the TT, years spent at school were found to influence performance and scores must be corrected according to years spent in schooling. On the plus-minus score, a corrected score of 18.35 was found to classify 8 per cent of the aphasic group as having normal expressive abilities. This constitutes a hit rate of 92 per cent for aphasic subjects. Between 10 per cent and 15 per cent of the brain-damaged, but non-aphasic, group were classified as having some degree of expressive language impairment (a hit rate of between 85 per cent and 90 per cent). These hit rates were observed to be superior to a series of standard expressive language tests administered to the aphasic and non-aphasic brain-damaged groups. With the weighted score, a cutting score of 54 classified 18 per cent of aphasic subjects as non-aphasic and 15 per cent of non-aphasic left hemisphere-damaged subjects as aphasic; hit rates of 82 per cent and 85 per cent respectively.

Therapeutic Implications

Investigations into the value of the TT as a basis for rehabilitation of comprehension deficit have demonstrated so far that qualitative analysis of TT performances can provide the clinician with information upon which to base treatment. Studies have shown, for instance, that shape (particularly 'square') tends to produce more errors than colour or size (De Renzi and Vignolo, 1962; Holland and Sonderman, 1974; Mack and Boller, 1979).

Holland and Sonderman conducted a study of a treatment programme based on the TT format. Using a programmed instruction approach, they attempted to train 24 aphasic patients on shape, size, colour and the command structure of the TT. Subjects were pre-tested and post-tested on the TT and selected subtests of the Minnesota. Subjects' scores on the pre-treatment TT fell into two groups with one group achieving scores between 21 and 31 (the 'high' group) and the other group achieving scores between 2 and 13 (the 'low' group). Most subjects showed some gains on post-test with the high group showing statistically significant improvement. Although 9 of the low group (N = 14) made gains, as a group the improvement was insignificant. No statistically reliable change was noted in Minnesota scores for either group.

The conclusion of this study seems to be that patients with less severe comprehension deficits may benefit from systematic 'token test training' (in this study, those with scores above 21 items correct), but the more severe (item scores below 13) will benefit less. The failure of patients as a whole to make significant improvements on the Minnesota may indicate, as Holland and Sonderman conclude, that subjects were unable to generalise to other language tasks. However, it may also reflect a lack of sensitivity to change in the Minnesota test. The treatment programme appeared to be particularly effective in improving performance of some complex TT commands in Part V like negation 'no' (item 16), 'instead' (item 17) and 'away from' (item 7). There were indications also that providing a written version of the auditory command significantly improves performance.

A similar study by West (1973) used real objects in a systematic programme based on the TT format. Significant improvement in TT scores are reported for four out of five subjects as well as generalisation to Minnesota results. Salvatore (1975) and Liles and Brookshire (1975) have examined the effects of inserting pauses of varying lengths between TT stimuli. Salvatore noted improved TT scores with pauses of two to five seconds. Holland and Whitney (1979) comment that this approach could be developed into a systematic treatment programme to improve comprehension where pauses are gradually reduced. Code (forthcoming) in an attempt to train the undamaged right hemisphere of a stabilised Wernicke's aphasic patient, adapted the assessment method used by Albert and Bear (1974) by presenting two and three digits and two and three words with gradually reducing pauses between them via a dichotic listening treatment programme. Large improvements in comprehension and retention of digits were noted with modest improvements in TT and PICA scores.

The potential of the Reporter's Test as a basis for planning remediation has yet to be explored. However, the reported qualitative power of the test would suggest that it may be particularly useful for the clinician planning treatment by revealing and measuring anomia, phonemic and semantic paraphasia, circumlocution, perseveration and the whole range of expressive symptoms which characterise encoding aspects of aphasia. The detection and quantification of the widely accepted parameters of aphasic non-fluency – phrase length, disturbed prosody, speech rate, telegraphic speech, etc. – with the RT should help the clinician. The test's apparent superiority to less controlled methods of eliciting and measuring expressive language should provide the clinician with the necessary information to assess the relative contribution of each parameter to an individual patient's particular problems with fluency.

It may be that, as with the TT, programmes might be designed based on the format and structure of the Reporter's Test aimed at remediation of a patient's particular areas of deficit on the test. Further control evaluation would then be necessary to establish whether any improvement had generalised.

Related Research

Knowledge of what it is that the TT is assessing in aphasic patients is uncertain. Boller, Kim and Mack (1977) in their review of research carried out over the last decade with the TT conclude that 'the reasons aphasics tend to perform poorly in comparison with groups of other patients and with control groups is not clear' (p. 29). This is probably due to the fact that knowledge of what constitutes comprehension impairment in various types of aphasia is so limited. Lesser (1974; 1976; 1979) has produced evidence to suggest that most of the commands of the TT have information content of six items which may be beyond the short term memory span of aphasic patients. This factor may influence scores rather than comprehension of speech *per se*. Lesser (1976) also suggests that the ordering and sequencing of elements is impaired in aphasia and that this will be reflected in a patient's score, as well as difficulties in visual and gestural sequencing. She considers that the TT has obvious clinical relevance as a screening procedure for the detection of aphasia, but there is no justification for drawing conclusions about the linguistic complexity of particular words or sentence structures from performance on the TT, when performance probably has more to do with non-linguistic factors.

Needham and Swisher (1972) in a comparison of the original TT, the understanding section of the FCP and the comprehension section of an aphasia battery, confirmed that the TT was best at revealing mild impairments in comprehension but less useful for the assessment of severely impaired patients due to the limited number of responses obtained from such patients. The revised version of the TT discussed above, with its new easier first section, should be more useful in assessing the more severely impaired.

The test-retest reliability of the original TT has been examined by Gallaher (1979) who tested 30 aphasic subjects three times over an eight day period. High test-retest reliability was noted where correlations between test days ranged from +0.91 to +0.98. There did not appear to be any learning effect over the three testings, as differences between test days were below significance. Furthermore, the results of the analysis indicated that 'the day to day performances of aphasic patients are reliable regardless of time since onset' (p. 39). Fifteen of the subjects from the total 30 were tested less than three months post-onset.

Appraisal

The revised TT and the RT taken together constitute a potentially useful battery to the clinician for determining levels of functioning in comprehension and expression, and as a basis for planning remediation, especially for milder forms of aphasia which may be undetected by more conventional assessments. The work reviewed above suggests that treatment could follow the TT and RT format with modifications to variables like time between separate elements of commands or stimuli and length and complexity of commands or stimuli. No doubt future investigations with the RT will examine memory and intellectual components of the assessment, as well as its potential for detecting and measuring agraphia.

Conclusion

The assessment procedures discussed above have included comprehensive batteries like the Boston, Minnesota and PICA, which were designed to detect and measure linguistic impairment across modalities and at all levels of language use, and other tests designed to evaluate specific aspects of aphasic disturbance like the FCP, TT and RT.

Most of the tests examined have been shortened, and in the case of some tests several shortened versions are now available. The originators of the tests are, for the most part, concerned that test reliability suffers as a result of shortening, but the studies cited above indicate that reliability does not suffer, and that much redundancy exists in the longer comprehensive batteries. However, the short forms of the Minnesota and PICA reviewed above were not actually administered as short forms in the studies reported, but were developed from analyses of administering full versions. Comparisons of results from separately administered short and full forms would appear to be necessary to confirm the high positive correlations reported.

In the final instance the clinician has to decide between a shorter, more convenient version of a test, or a longer, more comprehensive assessment. It would seem that for diagnosis and prediction of outcome, a reliable short version would suffice; but the clinician will require the detailed information provided in the comprehensive battery, which assesses a broad sample of language behaviour, in order to plan treatment for specific areas of deficit.

In recent years there has been a growing awareness of the importance of non-verbal aspects of communication in aphasia therapy, and it would appear that more comprehensive assessment of these factors should be included in aphasia tests.

Each of the tests examined above has its strengths and weaknesses for the clinician concerned with planning and carrying out treatment, and probably most clinicians would want to have a selection of tests available to them. These tests will be chosen to meet their own particular clinical requirements and individual preferences.

6 APPLYING BEHAVIOURISTIC TECHNIQUES

Chapter Outline

The use of behaviouristic techniques in language therapy is discussed. Special emphasis is placed on the practical problems of assessing language from a behaviouristic standpoint and on implementing suitable treatment techniques. A selective review of research with children and adult aphasics is presented, and it is concluded that the application of behaviouristic techniques is effective in a variety of cases. The possibility of using friends and family in therapy and the importance of adapting treatment to the subject's natural environment are raised for further discussion.

Introduction

Behaviouristic techniques are based on the simple assumption that language is to some extent learned and can therefore be taught. This notion mentioned earlier in Chapter 2 is supported in part by research into the use of behaviouristic techniques in language therapy, some of which will be reviewed in this chapter. Furthermore, as Müller (1980) points out, if behaviouristic techniques are demonstrably effective, this will direct future research towards evaluating the best ways of utilising the known facts about learning.

In conducting remediation, therapists often used a variety of behaviouristic techniques to shape the language behaviour of their patients. At one level this may simply entail the spontaneous use of reinforcement or imitation, techniques which seem to be used by almost every therapist or teacher. More sophisticated applications of behaviouristic techniques involve the use of structured programmes which have to be implemented in a stricter and more rigid manner. Whereas some therapists and teachers consciously choose structured approaches a vast majority appear to use behaviouristic techniques without having deliberated in any precise way on their implementation. There is then, a need for some of the implicit assumptions concerning behaviouristic techniques to be made more explicit.

Sloane and MacAulay (1968) present a clear exposition of the theoretical basis for behaviouristic techniques in the first chapter of their excellent book of readings. They note that the main emphasis is placed on the behavioural consequences of the language deficiency itself and not on some 'underlying' cause. Hence, speech and language are seen as developing out of the current behaviour of an individual in conjunction with the environmental antecedents and consequences of this behaviour. Therefore, remediation is directed towards modifying the environment in such a way as to change speech and language behaviour. As Sloane and MacAulay point out, this approach has two major advantages. First, the deficiency is expressed in terms of observable behaviour; and secondly, emphasis is placed on environmental rather than constitutional factors, this having direct implications for remediation.

Assessment and Remediation: Practical Considerations

Including the edited text by Sloane and MacAulay (1968) and in particular the paper by Johnston and Harris (1968) on assessment, there are a number of excellent guides to implementing behaviouristic techniques. Three relatively short papers are highly recommended. Kiernan (1974) provides a comprehensive analysis of behaviour modification which includes details of all the major concepts. These are discussed in detail by Howlin (1980) with reference to children, and by Sidman, Stoddard, Mohr and Leicester (1971) for aphasic patients. This section of the chapter will focus in more general terms on some of the practical considerations in applying behaviouristic techniques to language therapy.

In beginning therapy the starting point is an objective assessment of the patient's language in order to select *target behaviours*. As suggested by Howlin (1980) standardised tests, such as the Reynell discussed earlier, may be helpful in identifying children's specific language difficulties. However, from a behaviouristic perspective the most important aspect of assessment is undertaking what is termed a *functional analysis*. This is intended to identify the relationship between an individual's observed language behaviours and the environment within which these behaviours are elicited and thereby controlled.

Yule (1980) suggests that a functional analysis should consist of a systematic inquiry into the antecedents, characteristics and the consequences of any piece of behaviour. The LARSP discussed earlier could form the basis for this; by carefully observing and recording the context in which the speech sample was obtained, more detailed information can be built up. For example, it may be found that certain syntactical errors result from a father's, rather than a mother's, questioning and that the former usually results in the child making even more errors.

A similar analysis could be undertaken in assessing attention control along the lines suggested by Cooper *et al.* (1978) and discussed earlier (see Figure 3.4). A more thorough analysis of the antecedents of the development of attention control, such as the role of the mother or the type of stimuli used, is important. Similarly, by observing the effects of attention control, such as which factors help maintain it, a more complete diagnostic profile could be built up. Using this approach it should be possible to programme therapy more accurately.

Overall, functional analysis may provide more information of a qualitative nature than some of the assessment techniques discussed in earlier chapters. There are two general reasons for this. First, assessment is *naturalistic* and where possible undertaken in the everyday environment of the patient; and secondly, the patient's language is assessed in relationship to a variety of situations, including the way others respond and interact to the behaviour in question. This approach then, offers a wider perspective on assessment.

Having identified target behaviours and established *baseline* measures of performance prior to therapy, it is then possible to link specified language behaviours to controlling features in the environment in order to implement treatment. The main techniques used for children and adults are modelling or imitation, prompting, fading and reinforcement.

In some situations the use of modelling and imitation is sufficient in itself to elicit language. Peterson (1968) suggests that imitation can be used in the remediation of speech problems providing careful consideration is given to the use of reinforcement and to whether or not the behaviour is generalised in the absence of the model. Similarly the work of Elbert and McReynolds (1978) discussed in Chapter 2 emphasises the importance of imitation.

In many cases, imitation can be supplemented by the use of *shaping* and *fading* (Tsoi and Yule, 1980). Shaping consists of building up approximations to the desired sound by providing prompts and positively reinforcing correct behaviour. This forms the basis for a great deal of relatively simple articulation work which could be based for example on the Edinburgh Articulation Test discussed in Chapter 2. After this target behaviour has been established, the controlling factors such as prompts and reinforcement, are gradually faded so that the desired behaviour can be put under the control of the subject rather than the environment.

The most important factor affecting the use of behaviouristic techniques is the concept of reinforcement. Reinforcers serve to link an individual's behaviour with the environment and do not exist in isolation. Considerable care must be exercised in selecting the most appropriate reinforcer and delivering it in the most effective manner. The type of reinforcers used can range from food, such as sweets or chocolate, to general social reinforcement such as smiling and hugging. Adults with acquired language disorders may respond well to praise, but careful attention must be paid by the therapist to presenting this information by using verbal and non-verbal cues.

Hemsley and Carr (1980), in a most useful paper, point out that there are at least four important rules in presenting reinforcement. First, it should be entirely contingent on the desired behaviour actually occuring. Secondly, it should be presented as soon as the desired behaviour occurs, although it can be suggested that intermittent reinforcement might be more effective in some cases. Thirdly, reinforcement must be administered in a consistent fashion and finally, it is crucial that the subject is aware that reinforcement has been given. A further important point noted by Kiernan (1974) is that satiation can be avoided by the use of multiple reinforcers, but in a successive, that is one after the other, rather than in a simultaneous fashion.

This discussion of prompting and reinforcement is very interesting in the light of the Porch Index of Communicative Ability (see Chapter 5) which includes cueing in administering and scoring the test. It may be that more consideration should be given to administering tests with and without reinforcement and cueing in order to build up some idea of the therapeutic strategies which may be most appropriate for an individual patient. Those who perform better with prompting may in fact respond better to a behaviouristic approach to treatment, although as yet there is little evidence to support this.

The behaviouristic techniques already discussed are all used to some extent in the most structured form of therapy available, that of programmed instruction. Costello (1977) in a detailed analysis of the therapeutic implications of programmed instruction, refers to it as a systematically designed plan which specifies in detail the behaviours required of both the teacher and the learner. This approach is broadly based on the techniques derived from programmed learning and in particular programmed texts and teaching machines.

There are certain principles underlying programmed instruction which need to be considered. First, they are designed specifically to enable patients to work at their own pace, often alone and without the help of a therapist or teacher. Secondly, reinforcement should be immediate, for correct responses and errors are thereby minimised by breaking down the material into extremely small and easy steps. Thirdly, through the use of modelling and prompting successive approximations to the desired response can be built up, and finally, these cues should then be faded so that the ultimate product of the programme generalises and occurs naturally in the individual's own environment. As might be predicted, the development of such programmes is very costly in terms of time and often has to be restricted to a specific component of language, such as a selected verb.

In summary there are at least seven major practical considerations in implementing behaviouristic techniques in a systematic manner:

(i) *baseline* measures of the speech or language behaviour in question must be identified through undertaking a *functional analysis;*
(ii) the *target* behaviours must be objectively defined;
(iii) the techniques to be used need careful specification, and reinforcers must be selected which are appropriate to the patient's natural environment;
(iv) *generalisation* should be built into the programme and individuals concerned with the patient need to be involved;
(v) prompts and cues should gradually be *faded* and a schedule of reinforcement introduced which is similar to that which patients may find in their natural environment;
(vi) systematic assessment should be on-going and be seen as part of the programme; and
(vii) the *target* behaviours should be assessed in the patient's natural environment.

By considering these factors, it should be possible to implement behaviouristic techniques in a more systematic, explicit and effective manner.

Selected Research

Children

There are a number of reviews of research evaluating the effectiveness of behaviouristic techniques with children. Yule, Berger and Howlin (1975) have suggested that there was sufficient evidence to warrant further examination of the techniques outlined above, and in an extensive review of behavioural approaches to language training for the severely retarded, Snyder, Lovitt and Smith (1975) concluded that performance could be improved through the application of systematic instructional techniques and careful reinforcement. More recently, Margolies (1977) in a review of behaviouristic approaches to treating early infantile autism, argues that language is an appropriate target for this form of remediation.

In order to illustrate how behaviouristic approaches can be used effectively in a variety of situations, consideration will be given to four particular programmes covering a range of language disorders. The work of Lovaas (1977) will be discussed to illustrate how this technique can be used with autistic children having severe communication problems. A study conducted by Gray and Fygetakis (1968) with dysphasic children based on programmed learning will be reviewed, and two studies with developmentally delayed children will be examined to illustrate how operant conditioning can be applied to learning pronouns, verbs (Hegde and Gierut, 1979) and vocabulary (Cottrell, Montague, Farb and Thorne, 1980).

The programmes implemented by Lovaas (1977) and his colleagues were designed for autistic children having absolutely no discernible knowledge of language. This involved the use of fundamental behaviouristic techniques to teach the very rudiments of language. Programme I, for example, was simply aimed at training a child to discriminate between two sounds. Even with the constant use of reinforcement and systematic shaping of behaviour, it took on average 26 days of training for 7 hours a day to establish the desired patterns of behaviour.

A more advanced programme focused on elementary grammatical skills such as transforming simple verbs from the present to the past tense and learning plurals. It should be noted that regular verbs and plurals were taught in the same manner as the irregular ones. This was because the children were not able to assimilate and generalise to any great extent the rules of language.

The difficulties of evaluating the effectiveness of this kind of approach have been discussed elsewhere (Müller, 1980). If the communicative abilities of the autistic children are compared before and after therapy, it can be argued that the programmes were successful. Yet given the level of performance reached and the time it took, it can be suggested that the children may only have acquired specific responses rather than any understanding of language. However, even this relatively low level of performance may have given parents a great deal of encouragement, and this may be the only meaningful way to evaluate the effectiveness of this approach.

Gray and Fygetakis (1968) used an approach which was designed to combine behaviour therapy within the structure of programmed learning. This they termed 'programmed conditioning'. Their study used six children of approximately 5 years of age with a mean expressive language age of almost 3½ years. General conduct was brought under control by the use of tokens which were gained for good, and lost for bad, behaviour. Once this had been established, a specific programme was worked out in accordance with the information gained from an initial language assessment.

Each programme was worked out in detail to cover the development of a certain aspect of language. One specific programme, for example, designed to teach the verb 'is' consisted of seventeen discrete steps. Further details are provided covering the use of modelling, the schedules of reinforcement, progression to the next stage, the presentation of material, the forms of response which are acceptable and the estimated complexity of each step. Reinforcement was provided through a combination of tokens which could be traded in for small toys and social approval.

The results of this study suggested that programmed conditioning was effective in remedying a variety of language deficits. It was further noted that the target response of successfully completed programmes was often used by the children when playing. This generalisation indicated that the children had a greater understanding of language than was the case in the studies undertaken by Lovaas. It was also found that volunteers were able to use the system under the guidance of the experimenters. This is an important finding, bearing in mind the time taken in implementing such programmes. For example, fifteen 30 minute sessions were needed to teach the use of the word 'is'. Without help, this may just not be feasible in most clinical settings, despite the positive results reported in this study.

The use of operant techniques to train a language delayed boy to use the verb form 'are' and the three pronouns 'she', 'him' and 'he', are reported by Hegde and Gierut (1979). Baseline measures for all four target behaviours were recorded and pictures used to elicit the desired words. This was reinforced by providing food and tokens which could be traded in for free play. Incorrect responses were punished by showing the boy a card with 'no' written on it and by avoiding eye-contact. Modelling and imitation were used where appropriate.

It was found that all four target behaviours were successfully taught using these techniques. In addition, the young boy was able to use these responses when presented with new pictures depicting similar situations.

This finding led to the claim that there was a 100 per cent generalisation of trained responses to untrained stimuli. To test this fully, it would be necessary to see whether these language forms were used spontaneously in the young boy's natural environment.

A similar approach was used by Cottrell, Montague, Farb and Thorne (1980) to teach vocabulary to a young girl with Down's syndrome. This study included a novel approach towards assessing generalisation. The first eight words of the unrevised Wechsler Intelligence Scale for Children (see Chapter 1) were selected and training undertaken only on words of the same semantic class to see whether this generalised to the original word. For example, 'bicycle' was the first WISC word used and training was directed towards 'bus', 'plane' and 'boat', all words of the same semantic class.

Cottrell *et al.* (1980) found that behaviouristic techniques were successful in teaching the young girl to identify and define selected words. More importantly, they found that training on selected words generalised to other words in the same semantic class. This finding suggests that it is not necessary to teach the meaning of every word for vocabulary to increase. These results were confirmed in two further case studies.

In summary, the above studies suggest that it can be concluded that behaviouristic techniques are relatively effective in modifying language behaviour in children. This appears to be the case particularly when working with the lower order and more specific aspects of language. The difficulty in assessing the extent to which selected target behaviours can be generalised is evident and it is not easy to arrive at any definitive conclusion. However, as an approach towards remediating children's language, providing the clinician has sufficient time, these techniques might be seen as complementary to some of those examined in the earlier chapters.

Adult Aphasia

There are relatively few investigations into the effectiveness of behaviouristic techniques with aphasic adults, as is evident in a review by Seron, Van Der Linden, and Van Der Kaa-Delvenne (1978). Three studies using this general approach will be considered, two of which may be indicative of future trends towards using computer assisted treatment.

Holland and Harris (1968) present a detailed case study illustrating the use of programmed instruction. The patient was a young intelligent and well motivated male, whose symptoms although not too severe, caused considerable problems. Treatment lasted for 8 months and consisted of 5 hours a week of programmed instruction with a therapist, 2 hours a week group therapy and a further 10 hours a week at home of self-instruction. The therapists suggested that therapy for aphasics, was a process of re-establishing language, and that learning one programme in detail would generalise to similar and related material.

Each programme is described in detail in the original paper. The first programme used consisted of a series of 'usage tasks' designed to introduce simple sentences such as 'I sit at the table on a chair'. Although this programme was completed successfully, it indicated that the patient had problems in retaining and comprehending auditory information. The next two programmes were designed to rectify this. A home based programme on sensory functions designed to remediate 'semantic reversal problems', such as nose for mouth, was then introduced. Finally, two programmes designed to improve spelling were used.

The results of this study show that the patient improved. His conversational speech increased to a much higher level and included longer sentences and a greater variety of words, his writing improved and he was better able to describe pictures. This was in addition to successfully completing the programmes. It is concluded that programmed instruction is a potentially useful approach, despite the time taken in designing and administering programmes. However, in their otherwise favourable review of this study, Seron *et al.* (1978) note that despite the reported progress, there is no way of telling whether another remedial method would not have been as effective.

A more recent report by Culton and Ferguson (1979) describes the development and application of five automated language programmes with seven aphasic patients. All were assessed with the Porch Index of Communicative Abilities (see Chapter 5) and classified as follows: 4 were 'moderate', 2 were 'marked' and 1 was 'severe'.

The training programmes included teaching and problem solving activities. In one series for example, the first frame consisted of an auditory stimulus, such as 'The boy eats'; the second presented the auditory stimulus again with a picture; and the final frame repeated the auditory stimulus with four pictures, in this case including one of a boy eating. The patient was required to select the picture which matched the auditory input.

The effectiveness of the training programme was assessed by a test which contained the same linguistic structures, but not the same vocabulary combinations as the training items. Pre- and post-training scores were recorded. It was found that the subjects solved a significantly greater number of linguistic problems on the post- as compared to the pre-test. Consequently, it was concluded that the subjects' comprehension of the structures contained in the programmes had improved as a result of the automated training procedure. Although it took an estimated ten times longer to prepare the materials than might normally be the case, Culton and Ferguson note that the materials can be used with a large number of patients which is considered to be one of the main advantages of programmed training.

The third study to be discussed by Seron, Deloche, Moulard and Rousselle (1980), evaluated the use of computer based therapy for the treatment of aphasic subjects with writing disorders. Five patients with varied communicative impairments made up the sample. The subjects typed words as they were dictated to them. Each correct letter typed was displayed on a screen, providing immediate reinforcement for the patients.

The effectiveness of the programme was assessed as in the previous study by the use of a pre- and post-test, which was handwritten rather than typed. This was given on completing the programme and again after six weeks. In the first post-test there was a marked decrease in the total number of words in which at least one error was made and in the total number of errors. Although after six weeks there was some overall deterioration, performance was still better than on the pre-test. This was despite the fact that one subject got worse due to becoming depressed. Of particular interest was that the training procedure which consisted of typing, appeared to have generalised to handwriting, although there was no evidence to show whether this was the case outside the testing situation.

These few studies strongly suggest that behaviouristic techniques can be applied in a variety of situations with aphasic patients. The most difficult problem would appear to be that of having sufficient time to spend in writing and designing detailed programmes, and in some instances in implementing intensive therapy. However, with the advent of computers and 'chips technology', the potential to expand work in this area is enormous. Hopefully, there will be further studies in the future to evaluate more thoroughly the therapeutic implications of behaviouristic approaches to aphasia therapy.

Conclusion

From this selective review of studies, it can be concluded that the application of behaviouristic techniques can be effective in a variety of cases. The main difficulty in evaluating the efficacy of these techniques, is that of assessing whether learning generalises to the patient's natural environment. This involves ensuring that the reinforcement used is appropriate to the patient's social world, and that further assessment is undertaken in naturalistic settings. A further implication is that therapy itself might need to be implemented not in the classroom or the clinic, but in the home or where the subject feels most comfortable. However these problems are common to different levels of generalisation discussed in previous chapters, including for example the work of Ingram (1976), Cooper *et al.* (1978) and Hodson (1978).

This conclusion inevitably leads to the suggestion that in some instances therapy might best be undertaken by the family or close friends. As Heifetz (1977) and Callias (1980) have pointed out, behaviouristic techniques can be taught to, and implemented by, non-professionals especially parents. Given the importance of generalisation and the need to implement treatment in realistic settings, it may be that developments in language assessment and remediation lie outside the traditional domains of schools, hospitals and clinics. This proposition will now be considered in more detail.

7 NATURALISTIC CONSIDERATIONS

Chapter Outline

Recent developments in naturalistic approaches towards planning therapeutic strategies are discussed. The therapeutic rationale for working in the patient's own environment is considered and the role of friends and family examined. Selected research relating to children and aphasic patients is reviewed and the practical problems recognised. In conclusion, the notion of accountability is introduced and it is suggested that ultimately therapists and teachers accept full responsibility for their own decisions.

Introduction

This book has described and evaluated in considerable detail the links between assessment and remediation. It is hoped that this has been done without having lost sight of the main aim of remediation, that of generalising any improvement to the everyday world of the patient. Therapeutic change which is specific only to the clinical setting or is dependent upon the presence of the clinician, is of little value in helping the patient adjust to the real world. Consequently, it is important to consider the extent to which assessment and remediation can be related to the patient's natural environment.

In assessing language behaviour, a naturalistic approach would have to be based more on structured observation than standardised tests. This is clearly more subjective and involves considerable expertise on behalf of the therapist. Even video-taped material has to be interpreted and there is no guarantee that therapists will always be accurate in judging other people's behaviour. The time available also has to be taken into account. Naturalistic assessment is almost certain to take longer than the administration of most traditional test material.

Similarly, remediation is likely to be far more involved and complex despite the fact that it is often based upon simple behaviouristic techniques. There are two broad approaches therapists and teachers can take. One is simply to teach parents, family or friends specific techniques so that therapy continues outside the clinical situation, as in the work of Cooper *et al.* (1978) discussed earlier (see Chapter 3). The other is to direct therapy towards those in close contact with patients, in order to change their behaviour rather than that of the patients *per se*. The basic assumption of this approach is that the patient's problems are in fact caused by others, a radical departure from traditional remediation.

A naturalistic approach will involve teachers and therapists working in a very different way. Patients are no longer segregated into special categories and isolated from their natural environment. Instead, the clinicians will have to become more involved with the outside world of their patients and make more subjective judgements of the best way in which to conduct and evaluate therapy.

Therapeutic Rationale

In working with children it is not very difficult to justify a naturalistic approach towards therapy. There have been a number of studies investigating the role of the mother as a causal agent in children's acquisition of language. For example, Snow (1978) has suggested that in talking to their children, mothers create situations in which certain conditions are met to help establish effective communication. This is illustrated in the empirical work of Ratner and Bruner (1978). They suggest that simple appearance and disappearance games establish certain rules of taking turns which help children learn the conventions of conversation and how to communicate effectively with others. Similarly, Moerk (1976) has stressed the significance of interpersonal relationships between children and adults in the acquisition of language.

From a clinical perspective there have been a number of papers discussing the importance of naturalistic approaches. Mahoney (1975) has suggested that interpersonal factors may be causal in the development of language among mentally retarded and autistic children and similar arguments have been put forward by Snyder and McLean (1976) and by Brooks and Baumeister (1977). Beveridge and Brinker (1980) in an excellent review stress the importance of understanding the way in which retarded children interact with each other and establish reciprocal relationships with their teachers. These arguments clearly suggest that language remediation is more likely to be effective if implemented in the child's own environment.

This is clearly the case when working with bilingual children. It is not uncommon for language intervention techniques to be based on those strategies which adults normally adopt in speaking to children. An understanding of the bilingual situation from this naturalistic perspective would appear to be crucial. A further problem in a field as complex as bilingualism, is that few therapists actually have expertise in all the languages they might meet. As suggested earlier, this necessitates a team approach in the child's natural environment involving not only therapists but also close family. It would seem that naturalistic approaches can help teachers and therapists gain insight into the bicultural position of the children in their care, and help them to plan and implement more relevant treatment.

With aphasic patients the importance of taking into account their home and social background is obvious. This is often made more difficult by receiving imprecise information on the patient's premorbid mental state. Usually, the therapist has to build up a picture of the patient through interviewing and talking with close family and friends. Seron *et al.* (1978) however note that because this approach does not always provide reliable information, the patient's surroundings should be directly observed by the therapist. As discussed in Chapter 5, the Functional Communication Profile goes some way towards assessing a patient's ability to cope with real life. Furthermore, counselling of relatives is now an accepted part of working with aphasic patients, although there is little evidence to suggest that this is undertaken on the basis of naturalistic observation.

Similarly, friends and relatives can often be involved in implementing treatment. Although there is little systematic investigation of the effectiveness of this approach, Meikle, Wechsler, Tupper, Benenson, Butler, Mulhall and Stern (1979) have indicated that under the guidance of qualified therapists, trained volunteers are able to implement therapy. This form of treatment is usually undertaken in groups and is not really a substitute for working in naturalistic settings, although the work of Fawcus (forthcoming) does go someway towards remedying this.

Although the theoretical rationale for utilising naturalistic approaches in language assessment and remediation is well advanced, the practicalities of implementation have not as yet been solved. There are, however, a select number of studies which have been directed towards implementing this kind of approach. Some of these will be discussed in the following section.

Selected Research

Of particular interest are the results of a recent project on parental involvement with handicapped children, which resulted in an excellent series of books for non-professionals (Jeffree and McConkey, 1976; Jeffree, McConkey and Hewson, 1977a; 1977b). In a more recent research report, McConkey, Jeffree and Hewson (1979) examined the role of parents in extending the language development of their young mentally handicapped children. After training, the parents were made responsible for carrying out relevant language activities at home. It was found that the parents were successful in teaching their children not only to name objects but also to structure two-word sentences.

Another interesting series of studies with children has been undertaken by Seitz and her colleagues (Seitz and Hoekenga, 1974; Seitz and Riedell, 1974; and Seitz and Marcus, 1976). In these studies the parents were video-taped playing and talking with their children and a qualitative assessment made of their interactions. Therapy concentrated on teaching the parents how to elicit language from their children, rather than on the actual language problem itself. In general, the results of the studies were favourable and considerable improvement was found both in the way the parents reacted to their children and in the children's overall language performance.

More recent work by Clezy (1978; 1979) has resulted in a detailed language programme for parents and in particular for mothers to implement. It is argued that the mothers of 'language disordered' children are usually anxious, which leads to inappropriate 'interactive behaviours'. The first part of the treatment programme is designed to reduce this anxiety, by helping the mother employ appropriate strategies of reinforcement. She is then taught how to implement specially designed language programmes by adopting an interactive approach.

To help with this form of therapy, Cevette (1979) has developed a 'Reinforcement Profile', which enables clinicians to record their observations of the 'mother-child interchange'. It is suggested that this profile enables the mother to reflect critically upon her effectiveness as a therapist, and assists the supervising clinician in determining which procedures lead to improved language performance. The profile is simple to complete and would appear to have quite high reliability.

A similar approach has been adopted by Cheseldine and McConkey (1979). Seven Down's syndrome children took part in the study. All the children were at the one-two word stage of expressive language. Their parents were given a goal to work towards but were given no instruction on how to attain it. It was found that the most successful parents spontaneously altered their language and by using more selected target words in shorter utterances helped their children learn a greater number of these. A second study demonstrated that the less successful parents could be taught to modify their language which, in turn, improved the children's use of target words.

Although there is relatively little research on naturalistic approaches to aphasia therapy, the studies by Helmick *et al.* (1976) and Flowers *et al.* (1979) mentioned in Chapter 5, which found that spouses of aphasic patients tended to overestimate the patients' communicative skills, are indicative of current trends. The general criticisms made by Holland (1977) that the spouses' assessments may in fact have been more valid are interesting in the light of on-going work by Müller and Code (forthcoming). This is suggesting that inaccurate interpersonal judgements may in fact play a crucial role in therapy by providing motivation. Mulhall (1978) has suggested that enhancing the spouse's self-confidence is clearly beneficial to therapy and a method to produce graphical representations of the relationship is proposed. However, as yet there is insufficient evidence to come to any definite conclusions concerning naturalistic approaches to aphasia therapy.

Taken overall, these studies are indicative of a growing trend towards naturalistic language therapy. The difficulties in conducting research to evaluate the efficacy of this kind of approach are enormous. In particular, clinicians work with individual patients and tend not to be in a position to evaluate different therapeutic strategies. There is also, of course, the practical problem of conducting therapy in the patient's natural environment given that patients are usually seen only once or twice a week. However, the studies reviewed above do suggest that this approach is worthy of further consideration, and one can look forward to a growth of research in this area.

Conclusion

This concluding chapter has highlighted entirely different strategies for those involved in the assessment and remediation of language. A naturalistic approach extends, and to some extent alters, the traditional role of both teachers and therapists. By involving the patient's family and friends in therapy, the clinicians themselves become more exposed in that they have to be able to justify their therapeutic procedures to non-professionals. In this sense they will become more accountable to the general public.

Yet, set against this is a fixed organisational structure within which therapists and teachers have to work. This means that there are certain rules and procedures which have to be followed. It is then difficult to implement change in therapeutic planning, without to some extent confounding the administrative system, which has to fulfil its role given limited financial power.

Consequently, this presents a dilemma for clinicians. On the one hand they are accountable to their employers and on the other to their patients, and the two are not always in accord. What constitutes the better therapeutic approach for the patient may not always fit in with what is possible from an administrative viewpoint. Perhaps the only answer is for therapists and teachers to accept full therapeutic responsibility within the context of what in practice can be achieved.

REFERENCES

Abercrombie, D. (1967) *Elements of General Phonetics*. Edinburgh: Edinburgh University Press

Abudarham, S. (1980) 'The problems of assessing the linguistic potential of children with dual language systems and their implications for the formulation of a differential diagnosis' in M.F. Jones (ed.), *Language Disability in Children*. Lancaster: MTP

Albert, M. and Bear, D. (1974) 'Time to understand: a case study of word deafness with reference to the role of time in auditory comprehension' *Brain, 97*, 373-84

Anderson, J.D., Hess, R. and Richardson, K. (1980) 'Test-retest reliability of the Test for Auditory Comprehension of Language when it is used with mentally retarded children'. *J. Speech Hear. Dis., 45*, 195-9

Anderson, T., Bouveston, N. and Greenberg, F. (1971) 'Rehabilitation predictors in completed stroke'. *Final Report to the U.S. Social Rehab. Service*. Minneapolis: Kenny Rehab.Inst., American Rehab. Foundation

Anthony, A., Bogle, D., Ingram, T.T.S. and McIsaac, M.W. (1971) *The Edinburgh Articulation Test*. Edinburgh: Livingstone

Anthony, A. and McIsaac, M.W. (1970) 'Notes on patterns of development found by using the qualitative phonetic assessment sheet of The Edinburgh Articulation Test'. *Brit.J.Dis.Comm., 5*, 148-64

Aronson, M., Shatin, L. and Cook, J. (1956) 'A sociotherapeutic approach to the treatment of aphasic patients'. *J.Speech Hear.Dis., 21*, 352-64

Auckland, M.J.L. (1979) 'The Audiology Unit, Reading: a pre-school group' in D. Crystal, *Working with LARSP*. London: Edward Arnold

Bellugi-Klima, U. (1971) 'Some language comprehension tests' in C. Lavatelli (ed.), *Language Training in Early Childhood Education*. Urbana, Ill.: University of Illinois Press

Benson, D. (1967) 'Fluency in aphasia: correlation with radioactive scan localization'. *Cortex, 3*, 373-94

Beveridge, M. and Brinker, R. (1980) 'An ecological-developmental approach to communication in retarded children' in F.M. Jones (ed.), *Language Disability in Children*. Lancaster: MTP

Blackman, N. (1950) 'Group psychotherapy with aphasics'. *J. Nervous Ment. Diseases, III*, 154-63

Blood, G.W. and Greenberg, B.R. (1978) 'Normative data for the revised score sheet of The Test for Auditory Comprehension of Language'. *Lang. Speech Hear. Serv. Schools, 9*, 210-12

Bloom, L. and Lahey, M. (1978) *Language Development and Language Disorders*. New York: John Wiley

Boller, F., Kim, Y. and Mack, J. (1977) 'Auditory comprehension in aphasia' in H. Whitaker and H.A. Whitaker (eds.), *Studies in Neurolinguistics, Volume 3*. London: Academic Press

Boller, F. and Vignolo, L. (1966) 'Latent sensory aphasia in hemisphere damaged patients: an experimental study with the Token Test'. *Brain, 89*, 815-30

Boone, D. (1972) 'Review of the Porch Index of Communicative Ability' in O.K. Buros (ed.), *The Seventh Mental Measurements Yearbook*. Highland Park, NJ: Gryphon Press

Bowerman, M. (1973) *Early Syntactic Development*. London: Cambridge University Press

Brinton, J. (1979) 'Sentence repetition tasks compared with expressive language performance' in D. Crystal, *Working with LARSP*. London: Edward Arnold

Broadbent, D.E. (1971) *Decision and Stress*. London: Academic Press

Brooks, P.H. and Baumeister, A.A. (1977) 'A plea for consideration of ecological validity in the experimental psychology of mental retardation'. *Amer.J.Ment. Defic., 81*, 407-16

Brown, R. (1973) *A First Language: The Early Stages*. Cambridge, Mass.: Harvard University Press

Bruner, J.S. (1975) 'Language as an instrument of thought' in A. Davies (ed.), *Problems of Language and Learning*. London: Heinemann

Bush, W.J. and Giles, M.T. (1977) *Aids To Psycholinguistic Teaching*. Columbus, Ohio: Charles E. Merrill

Callias, M. (1980) 'Teaching parents, teachers and nurses' in W. Yule and J. Carr (eds.), *Behaviour Modification for the Mentally Handicapped*. London: Croom Helm

Carrow, E. (1973) *Test for Auditory Comprehension of Language*. Boston, Mass.: Teaching Resources Corporation

—— (1974) *The Carrow Elicited Language Inventory*. Boston, Mass.: Teaching Resources Corporation

Cevette, M.J. (1979) 'Analysis of mother-child interchange' in G. Clezy, *Modification of the Mother-Child Interchange in Language, Speech and Hearing*. London: Edward Arnold; Baltimore: University Park Press

Cheseldine, S. and McConkey, R. (1979) 'Parental speech to young Down's Syndrome children: an intervention study'. *Amer.J.Ment.Defic., 83*, 612-20

Clark, C., Crockett, D. and Klonoff, H. (1979a) 'Factor analysis of the Porch Index of Communicative Ability'. *Brain and Language, 7*, 1-7

—— (1979b) 'Empirically derived groups in the assessment of recovery from aphasia'. *Brain and Language, 7*, 240-51

Clezy, G. (1978) 'Modification of the mother-child interchange'. *Brit.J.Dis. Comm., 13*, 93-106

—— (1979) *Modification of the Mother-Child Interchange in Language, Speech and Hearing*. London: Edward Arnold

Code, C. (forthcoming) 'Hemispheric specialisation retraining in aphasia: possibilities and problems' in C. Code and D.J. Müller (eds.), *Aphasia Therapy*. London: Edward Arnold

Cooper, J., Moodley, M. and Reynell, J. (1974) 'Intervention programmes for pre-school children with delayed speech development'. *Brit.J.Dis.Comm., 9*, 81-91

—— (1978) *Helping Language Development. A Developmental Programme for Children with Early Language Handicaps*. London: Edward Arnold

—— (1979) 'The developmental language programme. Results from a five year study'. *Brit.J.Dis.Comm., 14*, 57-69

Cornelius, S. (1974) *A Comparison of the Elicited Language Inventory with Developmental Sentence Scoring Procedures in Assessing Language Disorders in Children*. Unpublished Master's Thesis, Austin: University of Texas

Costello, J.M. (1977) 'Programmed instruction'. *J.Speech Hear.Dis., 42*, 3-28

Cottrell, A.W., Montague, J., Farb, J. and Thorne, J.M. (1980) 'An operant procedure for improving vocabulary definition performances in developmentally delayed children'. *J.Speech Hear.Dis., 45*, 90-102

Croner, R.F. (1974) 'The development of language and cognition: the cognition hypothesis' in B. Foss (ed.), *New Perspectives in Child Development*. Harmondsworth: Penguin

Cruttenden, A. (1977) Review of 'Ingram, D. (1976 *Phonological Disability in Children*. London: Edward Arnold'. *Brit.J.Dis.Comm., 12*, 75-7

Crystal, D. (1979) *Working with LARSP*. London: Edward Arnold

Crystal, D., Fletcher, P. and Garman, M. (1976) *The Grammatical Analysis of Language Disability*. London: Edward Arnold

Culton, G.L. and Ferguson, P.A. (1979) 'Comprehension training with aphasic subjects: the development and application of five automated programs'. *J.Comm.Dis., 12*, 69-82

Daly, D.A. (1978) 'Elicited imitation in language assessment: a tool for formulating and evaluating treatment programs'. *J.Comm.Dis., 1*, 25-35

Davies, W.K. (1979) Review of 'Lloyd, G. (1977) *Deprivation and the Bilingual Child*. Oxford: Blackwell'. *Polyglot, 1*, fiche 2

De Renzi, E. and Faglioni, P. (1978) 'Normative data and screening power of a shortened version of the Token Test'. *Cortex, 14*, 41-9

De Renzi, E. and Ferrari, C. (1978) 'The Reporter's Test: a sensitive test to detect expressive disturbances in aphasics'. *Cortex, 14*, 279-93

De Renzi, E. and Vignolo, L. (1962) 'The Token Test: a sensitive test to detect receptive disturbances in aphasics'. *Brain, 85*, 665-78

Dever, R.B. (1977) Reviews of 'Crystal, D., Fletcher, P. and Garman, M. (1976) *The Grammatical Analysis of Language Disability*. London: Edward Arnold.' *J.Child Lang., 4*, 488-91

DiSimoni, F., Keith, R. Holt, D. and Darley, F. (1975) 'Practicality of shortening the Porch Index of Communicative Ability'. *J.Speech Hear.Res., 18*, 491-7

Dodd, B. (1978) Review of 'Ingram, D. (1976) *Phonological Disability in Children*. London: Edward Arnold'. *J.Ling., 14*, 89-122

Dulay, H.C., Hernández-Chávez, E. and Burt, M.K. (1978) 'The process of becoming bilingual' in S. Singh and J. Lynch (eds.), *Diagnostic Procedures in Hearing, Speech and Language*. Baltimore: University Park Press

Edwards, J.R. (1976) 'Disadvantage'. *Oideas, 16*, 53-58

—— (1979) *Language and Disadvantage*. London: Edward Arnold

Edwards, S., Ellams, J. and Thompson, J. (1976) 'Language and intelligence in dysphasia: are they related?' *Brit.J.Dis.Comm. 11*, 83-94

Egolf, D.B. and Chester, S.L. (1977) 'A comparison of aphasics' verbal performance in the language clinic with their verbal performance in other program areas of a comprehensive rehabilitation center'. *Rehabilitation Literature, 38*, 9-11

Eisenson, J. (1973) *Adult Aphasia: Assessment and Treatment*. Englewood Cliffs, NJ: Prentice-Hall

Elbert, M. and McReynolds, L.V. (1978) 'An experimental analysis of misarticulating children's generalization'. *J.Speech Hear. Res., 21*, 136-50

Elliott, C.D., Murray, D.J. and Pearson, L.S. (1978) *British Ability Scales*. Windsor: NFER

Ervin-Tripp, S. (1974) 'Is second language learning like the first?' *TESOL Quarterly, 8*, 111-27

Evesham, M. (1977) 'Teaching language skills to children'. *Brit.J.Dis.Comm., 12*, 23-9

—— (1980) 'Teaching language skills with the aid of the Illinois Test of Psycholinguistic Abilities' in F.M. Jones (ed.), *Language Disability in Children*. Lancaster: MTP

Farmer, A. and O'Connell, P. (1979) 'Neuropsychological processes in adult aphasia: rationale for treatment'. *Brit.J.Dis.Comm., 14*, 39-49

Farnham-Diggory, S. (1978) *Learning Disabilities*. London: Fontana/Open Books

Fawcus, M. (1964) 'Group therapy for the aphasic patient'. *Speech Path. and Therapy, 7, 30-6*

—— (forthcoming) 'Group therapy – a learning situation' in C. Code and D.J. Müller (eds.), *Aphasia Therapy*. London: Edward Arnold

Fenn, G. (1979) *Word Order Comprehension Test*. Windsor: NFER

Ferguson, C. (1968) 'Contrastive analysis and language development'. *Monograph Series on Language and Linguistics, Georgetown University, 21*, 101-10

Ferguson, C.A. (1959) 'Diglossia'. *Word, 15*, 325-40

Flowers, C.R., Beukelman, D.R., Bottorf, L.E. and Kelley, R.A. (1979) 'Family members' predictions of aphasic test performance'. *Aphasia, Apraxia, Agnosia, 1*, 18-26

Gallaher, A. (1979) 'Temporal reliability of aphasic performance on the Token Test'. *Brain and Language, 7*, 34-41

Geschwind, N. (1966) 'Discussion to paper by Wepman and Jones' in E. Carterette (ed.), *Brain Function: Volume 3*. Berkeley and Los Angeles: University of California Press

Goldman, R. and Fristoe, M. (1972) *Test of Articulation*. Circle Pines, Minn.: American Guidance Service Inc.

Goodglass, H. (ed.) (1978) *Selected Papers in Neurolinguistics*. München: Wilhelm Fink Verlag

Goodglass, H. and Geschwind, N. (1976) 'Language disorders (aphasia)' in E. Carterette and M. Friedman (eds.), *Handbook of Perception: Volume 7, Language and Speech*. London: Academic Press

Goodglass, H. and Kaplan, E. (1963) 'Disturbance of gesture and pantomime in aphasia'. *Brain, 86*, 703-20

—— (1972) *The Assessment of Aphasia and Related Disorders*. Philadelphia: Lea and Febiger

Goodglass, H., Klein, B., Carey, P. and Jones, K. (1966) 'Specific semantic word categories in aphasia'. *Cortex, 2*, 74-89

Goodglass, H., Quadfasel, F. and Timberlake, W. (1964) 'Phrase length and the type and severity of aphasia'. *Cortex, 1*, 133-53

Gray, B.B. and Fygetakis, L. (1968) 'Mediated language acquisition for dysphasic children'. *Behav.Res.Ther., 6*, 263-80

Greenberg, J.H. (1978) *Universals of Human Language* (4 vols.). Stanford, California: Stanford University Press

Grunwell, P.G. (1975) 'The phonological analysis of articulation disorders'. *Brit.J.Dis.Comm., 10*, 31-42

—— (1977) *The Analysis of Phonological Disability in Children*. Unpublished PhD Thesis: University of Reading

—— (1980) 'Developmental language disorders at the phonological level' in M.F. Jones (ed.), *Language Disability in Children*. Lancaster: MTP

Gumperz, J.J. and Hernández-Chávez, E. (1971) 'Cognitive aspects of bilingual communication' in W.H. Whitely (ed.), *Language Use and Social Changes*. London: Oxford University Press

Hammill, D.D. and Larsen, S.C. (1974) 'The effectiveness of psycholinguistic training'. *Excep.Child., 41*, 5-13

—— (1978) 'The effectiveness of psycholinguistic training: a re-affirmation of position'. *Except.Child., 44*, 402-14

Hammill, D.D. and Newcomer, P.L. (1980) 'Response to Maggiore's criticisms of the short form ITPA'. *Excep.Child., 46*, 434-8

Hanson, W. and Cicciarelli, A. (1978) 'The time, amount and pattern of language improvement in adult aphasics'. *Brit.J.Dis.Comm., 13*, 59-63

Hatfield, J.M. (1979) *Immigrant Children's Second Language Learning: The Application of Theory to Practice*. Unpublished Thesis presented in part fulfillment of Master of Applied Science Degree, University of Glasgow

Haugen, E. (1956) *Bilingualism in the Americas*. Alabama: University of Alabama Press

Hegde, M.N. and Gierut, J. (1979) 'The operant training and generalization of pronouns and a verb form in a language delayed child'. *J.Comm.Dis., 12*, 23-34

Heifetz, L.J. (1977) 'Behavioral training for parents of retarded children: alternative formats based on instruction manuals'. *Amer.J.Ment.Defic., 83*, 194-203

Heilporn, A. (1978) 'The socio-professional rehabilitation of neurologically handicapped people' in Y. Lebrun and R. Hoops (eds.), *The Management of Aphasia*. Amsterdam: Swets and Zeitlinger BV

Helmick, J.W., Watamori, T.S. and Palmer, J.W. (1976) 'Spouses' understanding of the communication disabilities of aphasic patients'. *J.Speech Hear.Dis.*, *41*, 238-43

Hemsley, R. and Carr, J. (1980) 'Ways of increasing behaviour-reinforcement' in W. Yule and J. Carr (eds.), *Behaviour Modification for the Mentally Handicapped*. London: Croom Helm

Hernández-Chávez, E. (1972) 'Early code separation in the second language Speech of Spanish-speaking children'. Unpublished Paper presented at the Stanford Child Language Forum, Stanford: University of Stanford

Hill, T.G. and Wallace, A.R. (1976) Review of 'Crystal, D.,Fletcher, P., and Garman, M. (1976) *The Grammatical Analysis of Language Disability*. London: Edward Arnold'. *Brit.J.Dis.Comm.*, *11*, 115-17

Hodson, B.W. (1978) 'A preliminary hierarchical model for phonological remediation'. *Lang.Speech Hear.Serv.Schools*, *9*, 236-40

Holland, A.L. (1977) 'Comment on "Spouses' understanding of the communication disabilities of aphasic patients" '. *J.Speech Hear.Dis.*, *42*, 307-8

Holland, A. and Harris, A. (1968) 'Aphasia rehabilitation using programmed instruction: an intensive case history' in H.N. Sloane, Jr and B.D. MacAulay (eds.), *Operant Procedures in Remedial Speech and Language Training*. Boston: Houghton Mifflin

Holland, A. and Sonderman, J. (1974) 'Effects of a program based on the Token Test for teaching comprehension skills to aphasics'. *J.Speech Hear.Res.*, *17*, 589-98

Holland, A. and Whitney, J. (1979) 'Non-diagnostic uses of the Token Test' in F. Boller and M. Dennis (eds.), *Auditory Comprehension: Clinical and Experimental Studies with the Token Test*. London: Academic Press

Howes, D. (1964) 'Application of the word-frequency concept to aphasia' in A.V. de Reuck and M. O'Conner (eds.), *Disorders of Language*. London: J. and A. Churchill

Howes, D. and Geschwind, N. (1964) 'Quantitative studies of aphasic language'. *Ass.Res.Nerv.Ment.Dis.*, *42*, 229-44

Howlin, P. (1980) 'Language training' in W. Yule and J. Carr (eds.), *Behaviour Modification for the Mentally Handicapped*. London: Croom Helm

Ingram, D. (1976) *Phonological Disability in Children*. London: Edward Arnold

Jeffree, D.M. and McConkey, R. (1976) *Let Me Speak*. London: Souvenir Press

Jeffree, D.M., McConkey, R. and Hewson, S. (1977a) *Teaching the Handicapped Child*. London: Souvenir Press

—— (1977b) *Let Me Play*. London: Souvenir Press

Jenkins, J., Jiménez-Pabón, E., Shaw, R. and Sefer, J. (1975) *Schuell's Aphasia in Adults*. New York: Harper and Row

Johnson, J.P., Winney, B.L. and Pederson, O.T. (1980) 'Single word versus connected speech articulation testing'. *Lang.Speech Hear.Serv.Schools*, *11*, 175-9

Johnson, M. and Tomblin, B. (1975) 'Reliability of developmental sentence scoring as a function of sample size'. *J.Speech Hear.Res.*, *18*, 372-80

Johnson, S. and Somers, H. (1978) 'Spontaneous and imitated responses in articulation testing'. *Brit.J.Dis.Comm.*, *13*, 107-16

Johnston, M. and Harris, F.R. (1968) 'Observation and recording of verbal behaviour in remedial speech work' in H.N. Sloane, Jr and B.D. MacAulay (eds.), *Operant Procedures in Remedial Speech and Language Training*. Boston: Houghton Mifflin

Jones, W.R. (1966) *Bilingualism in Welsh Education*. Cardiff: University of Wales Press

Karnes, M.B. (1972) *Goal Program: Language Development*. Springfield, Mass. Milton Bradley

Kerschensteiner, M., Poeck, K. and Brunner, E. (1972) 'The fluency-non fluency dimension in the classification of aphasic speech'. *Cortex, 8*, 233-47

Kertesz, A., Harlock, W. and Coates, R. (1979) 'Computer tomographic localization, lesion size, and prognosis in aphasia and nonverbal impairment'. *Brain and Language, 8*, 34-50

Khan, V.S. (1980) 'The Mother-tongue of linguistic minorities in multicultural England'. *J.Multiling. and Multicult.Dev., 1*, 71-88

Kiernan, C.C. (1974) 'Behaviour modification' in A.M. Clarke and A.D.B. Clarke (eds.), *Mental Deficiency: The Changing Outlook*. London: Methuen

Kirk, S.A. and Kirk, W.D. (1971) *Psycholinguistic Learning Disabilities: Diagnosis and Remediation*. Urbana, Ill.: University of Illinois Press

—— (1978) 'Uses and abuses of the ITPA'. *J.Speech Hear.Dis., 43*, 58-75

Kirk, S.A., McCarthy, J.J. and Kirk, W.D. (1968) *Examiner's Manual. Illinois Test of Psycholinguistic Abilities (revised edition)*. Urbana, Ill.: University of Illinois Press

Kirk, W.D. (1974) *Aids and Precautions in Administering the Illinois Test of Psycholinguistic Abilities*. Urbana, Ill.: University of Illinois Press

Lavine, S.B. (1978) 'The paired comparisons method of identifying developmental discrepancies with the ITPA'. *J.Learn.Dis., 11*, 506-10

Lee, L. (1969) *The Northwestern Syntax Screening Test*. Evanston: Northwestern University Press

—— (1974) *Developmental Sentence Analysis*. Evanston: Northwestern University Press

Leonard, L.B., Schwartz, R.G., Folger, M.K. and Wilcox, M.J. (1978) 'Some aspects of child phonology in imitative and spontaneous speech'. *J.Child Lang., 5*, 403-15

Lesser, R. (1974) 'Verbal comprehension in aphasia: an English version of three Italian tests'. *Cortex, 10*, 247-63

—— (1976) 'Verbal and non-verbal memory components in the Token Test'. *Cortex, 14*, 79-85

—— (1978) *Linguistic Investigations of Aphasia*. London: Edward Arnold

—— (1979) 'Turning tokens into things: linguistic and mnestic aspects of the initial sections of the Token Test' in F. Boller and M. Dennis (eds.), *Auditory Comprehension: Clinical and Experimental Studies with the Token Test*. London: Academic Press

Lieb, H-H. (1975) 'Universals of language: quandaries and prospects'. *Found. Lang,12*, 471-511

Liles, B. and Brookshire, R. (1975) 'The effects of pause time on auditory comprehension of aphasic subjects'. *J.Comm.Dis, 8*, 221-36

Lindholm, K.J. and Padilla, A.M. (1978) 'Language mixing in bilingual children'. *J.Child.Lang., 5*, 327-35

Lloyd, G. (1977) *Deprivation and the Bilingual Child*. Oxford: Blackwell

Lock, A. (1978) 'The emergence of language' in Lock, A. (ed.), *Action, Gesture and Symbol: The Emergence of Language*. London: Academic Press

Lovaas, O.I. (1977) *The Autistic Child: Language Development Through Behavior Modification*. New York: Irvington Publishers Inc.

Lowe, M. and Costello, A.J. (1976) *The Symbolic Play Test*. Windsor: NFER

Lund, K.A., Foster, G.E. and McCall-Perez, F.C. (1978) 'The effectiveness of psycholinguistic training, a re-evaluation'. *Excep.Child., 44*, 310-19

Luria, A.R. (1961) *The Role of Speech in the Regulation of Normal and Abnormal Behaviour*. Oxford: Pergamon

McConkey, R., Jeffree, D. and Hewson, S. (1979) 'Involving parents in extending the language development of their young mentally handicapped children'. *Brit.J.Dis.Comm.*, *14*, 203-18

McDonald, E.T. (1964) *Articulation Testing and Treatment: A Sensory-Motor Approach*. Pittsburgh: Stanwix House

McLaughlin, B. (1978) *Second Language Acquisition in Childhood*. New York: John Wiley

Macnamara, J. (1966) *Bilingualism and Primary Education: A Study of Irish Experience*. Edinburgh: Edinburgh University Press

—— (1972) 'Cognitive bases of language learning in infants'. *Psychol. Rev.*, *79*, 1-13

McNeill, D. (1970) *The Acquisition of Language*. New York: Harper and Row

Mack, J. and Boller, F. (1979) 'Components of auditory comprehension: analysis of errors in a revised Token Test' in F. Boller and M. Dennis (eds.), *Auditory Comprehension: Clinical and Experimental Studies with the Token Test*. London: Academic Press

Maggiore, R.P. (1978) 'Reliability of proposed short form of Illinois Test of Psycholinguistic Abilities'. *Excep.Child.*, *45*, 198-204

Mahoney, G.J. (1975) 'Ethological approach to delayed language acquisition'. *Amer.J.Ment.Defic.*, *80*, 139-48

Margolies, P.J. (1977) 'Behavioral approaches to the treatment of early autism: a review'. *Psychol.Bull.*, *84*, 249-64

Marinosson, G.L. (1974) 'Performance profiles of matched normal, educationally subnormal and severely subnormal children on the revised ITPA'. *J.Child Psychol. and Psychiat.*, *15*, 139-48

Martin, A.D. (1977) 'Aphasia testing: a second look at the Porch Index of Communicative Ability'. *J.Speech Hear.Dis.*, *42*, 547-62

Meikle, M., Wechsler, E., Tupper, A., Benenson, M., Butler, J., Mulhall, D. and Stern, G. (1979) 'Comparative trial of volunteer and professional treatments of dysphasia after stroke'. *Brit.Med.J.*, *2*, 87-9

Mikěs, M. (1967) 'Acquisition des catégoires grammaticales dans le language de l'enfant'. *Enfance*, *20*, 289-98

Miller, C.E. and Prutting, C.A. (1979) 'Inconsistencies across three language comprehension tests for specific grammatical features'. *Lang.Speech Hear. Serv.Schools*, *10*, 162-70

Miller, N. (1978) 'The bilingual child in the speech therapy clinic'. *Brit.J.Dis. Comm.*, *13*, 17-30

Milon, J.P. (1974) 'The development of negation in English by a second language learner'. *TESOL Quarterly*, *8*, 137-43

Mittler, P. (1976) 'Assessment for language learning' in P. Berry (ed.), *Language and Communication in the Mentally Handicapped*. London: Edward Arnold

Moerk, E.L. (1976) 'Processes of language teaching and training in the interactions of mother-child dyads'. *Child.Dev.*, *47*, 1064-78

Mulac, A., Prutting, C.A. and Tomlinson, C.N. (1978) 'Testing for a specific syntactic structure'. *J.Comm.Dis.*, *11*, 335-47

Mulhall, D.J. (1978) 'Dysphasic stroke patients and the influence of their relatives'. *Brit.J.Dis.Comm.*, *13*, 127-34

Müller, D.J. (1980) 'A critical evaluation of learning techniques in language therapy' in F.M. Jones (ed.), *Language Disability in Children*. Lancaster: MTP

—— (in press) 'On clinicians' undue respect for statistical significance'. *J.Learn. Dis.*

Müller, D.J. and Code, C. (forthcoming) 'Interpersonal perceptions of psychosocial adjustment to aphasia' in C. Code and D.J. Müller (eds.), *Aphasia Therapy*. London: Edward Arnold

Munro, S.M. (1979) 'Speech therapy for the bilingual child in Wales'. *Polyglot, 2*, fiche I

Naeser, M. and Hayward, R. (1978) 'Lesion localization in aphasia with cranial computed tomography and the Boston Diagnostic Aphasia Exam'. *Neurology, 28*, 545-51

Needham, L. and Swisher, L. (1972) 'A comparison of three tests of auditory comprehension for adult aphasics'. *J.Speech Hear. Dis., 37*, 123-31

Nelson, K. (1973) 'Structure and strategy in learning to talk'. *Monogr.Soc.Res. Child Dev., 38*, Serial No. 149

Newcomer, P. and Hammill, D. (1974) 'A short form of the Revised ITPA'. *J.Learn.Dis., 7*, 570-2

Newton, M.J., Thomson, M.E. and Richards, I.L. (eds.) (1979) *Readings in Dyslexia*. Wisbech: LDA

Oller, D.K., Jensen, H.T. and Lafayette, R.H. (1978) 'The relatedness of phonological processes of a hearing impaired child'. *J.Comm.Dis., 11*, 97-105

Paraskevopoulos, J.N. and Kirk, S.A. (1969) *The Development and Psychometric Characteristics of the Revised Illinois Test of Psycholinguistic Abilities*. Urbana, Ill.: University of Illinois Press

Paynter, E.T. and Bumpas, T.C. (1977) 'Imitative and spontaneous articulatory assessment of three-year-old children'. *J.Speech Hear.Dis., 42*, 119-25

Perera, K. (1980) Review of 'Crystal, D. (1979) *Working with LARSP*. London: Edward Arnold'. *Brit.J.Dis.Comm., 15*, 54-5

Peterson, R. (1968) 'Imitation: a basic behavioral mechanism' in H.N. Sloane, Jr and B.D. MacAulay (eds.), *Operant Procedures in Remedial Speech and Language Training*. Boston: Houghton Mifflin

Pfaff, C.W. (1979) 'Constraints on language mixing: intrasentential code-switching and borrowing in Spanish/English'. *Language, 55*, 291-318

Phillips, P. and Halpin, G. (1978) 'Language impairment evaluation in aphasic patients: developing more efficient measures'. *Arch.Phys.Med.Rehab., 59*, 327-30

Piaget, J. (1968) 'Language and thought from the genetic point of view' in J. Piaget, *Six Psychological Studies*. London: University of London Press

Poeck, K. and Hartje, W. (1979) 'Performance of aphasic patients in visual versus auditory presentation of the Token Test' in F. Boller and M. Dennis (eds.), *Auditory Comprehension: Clinical and Experimental Studies with the Token Test*. London: Academic Press

Porch, B. (1967) *The Porch Index of Communicative Ability. Volume 1: Theory and Development*. Palo Alto, California: Consulting Psychologists Press

—— (1971) *The Porch Index of Communicative Ability. Volume 2: Administration and Scoring*. Palo Alto, California: Consulting Psychologists Press

Porch, B., Collins, M., Wertz, R. and Friden, T. (1980) 'Statistical prediction of change in aphasia'. *J.Speech Hear.Res., 23*, 312-21

Powell, G., Bailey, S. and Clark, E. (1980) 'A very short version of the Minnesota Aphasia Test'. *Brit.J.Soc.Clin.Psych., 19*, 189-94

Powell, G., Clark, E. and Bailey, S. (1979) 'Categories of aphasia: a cluster-analysis of Schuell test profiles'. *Brit.J.Dis.Comm., 14*, 111-22

Prinz, P.M. (1980) 'A note on requesting strategies in adult aphasics'. *J.Comm. Dis., 13*, 65-73

Pyle, D.W. (1979) *Intelligence: An Introduction*. London: Routledge and Kegan Paul

Quirk, R., Greenbaum, S., Leech, G. and Svartvik, J. (1972) *A Grammar of Contemporary English*. London: Longman

Ratner, N. and Bruner, J. (1978) 'Games, social exchange and the acquisition of language'. *J.Child Lang., 5*, 391-401

Ravem, R. (1974) 'The development of Wh-questions in first and second language learners' in J.C. Richards (ed.), *Error Analysis: Perspectives on Second Language Learning*. London: Longman

Rees, N.S. and Shulman, M. (1978) 'I don't understand what you mean by comprehension'. *J.Speech Hear.Dis.*, *43*, 208-19

Reynell, J. (1969) 'A developmental approach to language disorders'. *Brit.J.Dis. Comm.*, *4*, 33-40

—— (1972) 'Language handicaps in mentally retarded children' in A.D.B. Clarke and M.M. Lewis (eds.), *Learning, Speech and Thought in the Mentally Retarded*. London: Butterworths

—— (1976) 'Assessment of language development' in B. Tanner (ed.), *Language and Communication in General Practice*. London: Hodder and Stoughton

—— (1977) *Manual for the Reynell Developmental Language Scales (revised)*. Windsor: NFER

Rondal, J.A. (1978) 'Developmental sentence scoring procedure and the delay-difference question in language development of Down's Syndrome children'. *Ment.Retard.*, *16*, 169-71

Ronjat, J. (1913) *Le Développement du Langage Observé chez un Enfant Bilingue*. Paris: Champion

Salvatore, A. (1975) 'An investigation of the effects of pause duration on sentence comprehension by aphasic subjects'. Paper presented at the Annual Meeting of the American Speech and Hearing Assoc., Washington, DC

Sampson, G. (1978) 'Linguistic universals as evidence for empiricism'. *J.Ling.*, *14*, 183-206

Sampson, O.C. (1976) 'Fifty years of dyslexia. A review of the literature 1925-75. II Practice'. *Res. in Ed.*, *15*, 39-53

Sattler, J.M. (1974) *Assessment of Children's Intelligence*. London: W.B. Saunders (revised reprint)

Schuell, H. (1957) 'A short examination for aphasia'. *Neurology*, *7*, 625-34

—— (1966) 'A re-evaluation of the short examination for aphasia'. *J.Speech Hear.Dis.*, *31*, 137-47

—— (1973) *Differential Diagnosis of Aphasia with the Minnesota Test*. Revised Edition. London: Oxford University Press

Schuell, H., Jenkins, J. and Carroll, J. (1962) 'A factor analysis of the Minnesota Test for Differential Diagnosis of Aphasia'. *J.Speech Hear.Res.*, *5*, 349-69

Seitz, S. and Hoekenga, R. (1974) 'Modeling as a training tool for regarded children and their parents'. *Ment.Retard.*, *12*, 28-31

Seitz, S. and Marcus, S. (1976) 'Mother-child interactions: a foundation for language therapy'. *Excep.Child.*, *42*, 445-9

Seitz, S. and Riedell, G. (1974) 'Parent-child interactions as the therapy target'. *J.Comm.Dis.*, *7*, 295-304

Seron, X., Deloche, G., Moulard, G. and Rousselle, M. (1980) 'A computer based therapy for the treatment of aphasic subjects with writing disorders'. *J.Speech Hear.Dis.*, *45*, 45-58

Seron, X., Van Der Linden, M. and Van Der Kaa-Delvenne, M. (1978) 'The operant school of aphasia rehabilitation' in Y. Lebrun and R. Hoops (eds.), *The Management of Aphasia*. Amsterdam: Swets and Zeitlinger BV

Sidman, M., Stoddard, L.T., Mohr, J.P. and Leicester, J. (1971) 'Behavioral studies of aphasia: methods of investigation and analysis'. *Neuropsychologia*, *9*, 119-40

Siegel, G.M., Winitz, H. and Conkey, H. (1963) 'The influence of testing instrument on articulatory responses of children'. *J.Speech Hear.Dis.*, *28*, 66-76

Silverman, F. (1974) 'The Porch Index of Communicative Ability (PICA): a psychometric problem and its solution'. *J.Speech Hear.Dis.*, *39*, 225-6

Sinclair-de-Zwart, H. (1969) 'Developmental psycholinguistics' in D. Elkind and J. Flavell (eds.), *Studies in Cognitive Development*. New York: Oxford University Press

Sloane, H.N. Jr and MacAulay, B.D. (eds.) (1968) *Operant Procedures in Remedial Speech and Language Training*. Boston: Houghton Mifflin

Sloat, C., Taylor, S.H. and Hoard, J.E. (1978) *Introduction to Phonology*. Englewood Cliffs, NJ: Prentice Hall

Slobin, D.I. (1973) 'Cognitive prerequisites for the development of grammar' in C.A. Ferguson and D.I. Slobin (eds.), *Studies of Child Language Development*. New York: Holt, Rinehart and Winston

Smith, M.E. (1935) 'A study of the speech of eight bilingual children of the same family'. *Child Dev.*, *6*, 19-25

Smith, N.V. (1973) *The Acquisition of Phonology: A Case Study*. London: Cambridge University Press

Snow, C. (1978) 'The conversational context of language acquisition' in R.N. Campbell and P.T. Smith (eds.), *Recent Advances in the Psychology of Language. Language Development and Mother-Child Interaction*. New York: Plenum Press

Snyder, L.K., Lovitt, T.C. and Smith, J.O. (1975) 'Language training for the severely retarded: five years of behavior analysis research'. *Excep. Child.*, *42*, 7-15

Snyder, L.K. and McLean, J.E. (1976) 'Deficient acquisition strategies: a proposed conceptual framework for analyzing severe language deficiency'. *Amer. J.Ment.Defic.*, *81*, 338-49

Somers, H. (1979) 'Using the computer to analyse articulation test data'. *Brit.J. Dis.Comm.*, *14*, 231-40

Sparks, R.W. (1978) 'Parastandardized examination guidelines for adult aphasia'. *Brit.J.Dis.Comm.*, *13*, 135-46

Spreen, O. and Benton, A. (1969) *Neurosensory Center Comprehensive Examination for Aphasia*. Victoria, BC: University of Victoria

Stampe, D. (1969) 'The acquisition of phonetic representation'. *Papers from the Chicago Linguistic Society, 5th Regional Meeting*, 443-54

Stevenson, J. and Richman, N. (1976) 'The prevalence of language delay in a population of three-year old children and its association with general retardation'. *Dev.Med. and Child Neurol.*, *18*, 431-41

Stoel-Gammon, C. (1980) 'Phonological analysis of four Down's Syndrome children'. *Applied Psycholinguistics*, *1*, 31-48

Stott, D.H. (1978) *Helping Children with Learning Difficulties. A Diagnostic Teaching Approach*. London: Ward Lock Educational

Taylor, M. (1965) 'A measurement of functional communication in aphasia'. *Arch.Phys.Med.Rehab.*, *46*, 101-7

Taylor, M. and Sands, E. (1965) 'Reliability measures of the Functional Communication Profile'. Paper presented at the Annual Meeting of the American Speech and Hearing Association, Chicago

Taylor-Sarno, M. (1969) *The Functional Communication Profile: Manual of Directions*. New York: New York University Medical Center

Terman, L.M. and Merrill, M.A. (1960) *Stanford-Binet Intelligence Scale*. London: George G. Harrap

Thompson, J. and Enderby, P. (1979) 'Is all your Schuell really necessary?' *Brit.J.Dis.Comm.*, *14*, 195-201

Thomson, M.E. and Grant, S.E. (1979) 'The WISC subtest profile of the dyslexic child' in M.J. Newton, M.E. Thomson and I.L. Richards (eds.), *Readings in Dyslexia*. Wisbech: LDA

Tierney, R.J. and Ames, W.S. (1978) 'Examining the diagnostic claims of the revised ITPA'. *J.Learn.Dis.*, *11*, 586-90

Tsoi, M. and Yule, W. (1980) 'Building up new behaviours – shaping, prompting and fading' in W. Yule and J. Carr (eds.), *Behaviour Modification for the Mentally Handicapped*. London: Croom Helm

Viaud, G. (1960) *Intelligence. Its Evolution and Forms*. London: Hutchinson

Vygotsky, L.S. (1962) *Thought and Language*. Cambridge, Mass.: MIT Press

Walker, S. and Williams, B. (1980) 'The response of a disabled elderly population to speech therapy'. *Brit.J.Dis.Comm.*, *15*, 19-29

Wallace, A. (1964) 'Comments on the scale for the measurement of language function'. *Speech Path. and Therapy*, *7*, 22-9

Wechsler, D. (1955) *Wechsler Adult Intelligence Scale*. New York: The Psychological Corporation

—— (1967) *Wechsler Pre-School and Primary Scale of Intelligence*. New York: The Psychological Corporation

—— (1974) *Wechsler Intelligence Scale for Children – Revised*. New York: The Psychological Corporation

Weiner, P.S. (1972) 'The perceptual level functioning of dysphasic children'. *J.Speech Hear. Res.*, *15*, 423-38

West, J. (1973) 'Auditory comprehension in aphasic adults'. *Arch.Phys. Med. and Rehab.*, *54*, 78-86

Whitaker, H.A. and Whitaker, H. (1979) 'Lexical, syntactic and semantic aspects of the Token Test: a linguistic taxonomy' in F. Boller and M. Dennis (eds.), *Auditory Comprehension: Clinical and Experimental Studies with the Token Test*. London: Academic Press

Yule, W. (1980) 'Identifying problems – functional analysis and observation and recording techniques' in W. Yule and J. Carr (eds.), *Behaviour Modification for the Mentally Handicapped*. London: Croom Helm

Yule, W., Berger, M. and Howlin, P. (1975) 'Language deficit and behaviour modification' in N. O'Connor (ed.), *Language, Cognitive Deficits, and Retardation*. London: Butterworths

NAME INDEX

SUBJECT INDEX

For Product Safety Concerns and Information please contact our EU representative GPSR@taylorandfrancis.com
Taylor & Francis Verlag GmbH, Kaufingerstraße 24, 80331 München, Germany

www.ingramcontent.com/pod-product-compliance
Lightning Source LLC
LaVergne TN
LVHW020626300926
849161LV00004B/626
* 9 7 8 0 8 1 5 3 7 9 6 3 8 *